Acknowledgements

To my contemporaries Sharon and Laurie, who share my passion for feet and my vision for possibility. Without their encouragement I may never have begun.

To my Irish friend Mary, who introduced me to the phrase: Once you hear something, you can't unhear it!

To my sister Carolyn, who has been a fountain of information since I opened my mind to possibility.

To my husband of forty-three years Robert, a true soul mate who has extended me in every way possible to achieve my potential.

To Kerri, Rachel, Carole and the others already mentioned, who gave me their time and expertise, anything is possible when you have a great team to support you.

To Fiona, the most helpful and accommodating person I could have ever wished to work with. The Universe knew I needed someone very special and led me to the perfect person.

To the thousands of feet I have worked on, thank you for the lessons you brought through my door.

To the people who owned those feet without whom none of this would have been possible, I extend my deepest gratitude. You have taught me so much that has changed my life.

I must also acknowledge the many people who gave their permission to use their stories. Whilst you may not have agreed with some of the conclusions I have drawn, I am grateful for the opportunity to include examples that may challenge, extend and encourage others. I trust that I have respected your privacy and confidentiality, and stayed within your requested parameters as I expanded some stories and abbreviated others.

Contents

About the Author

Since the age of twenty-five I have held the conviction that sickness is not meant to be part of everyday living. This idea seemed to be at odds with the world at large, for sickness was all around me.

I held fast to what I believed in and began to look for answers. For many years I only searched within the parameters of my church and religious beliefs and unknowingly, held a narrow band of focus and a mind that was closed to possibility.

When I began to study reflexology in 1998 I discovered a world I never knew existed and concepts that extended me as I had never been extended before. Almost everything I believed in to that point in my life began to change.

My search for the meaning of sickness and life in general began to move outside of all logic and comfortable parameters. I continued to look for the bigger picture, which wasn't always obvious and held on to a metaphysical connection to all things, which wasn't always shared by others.

While reflexology was the catalyst that opened my mind to possibility, the focus of my exploring, learning and experiences in more recent years has been directed to the esoteric, metaphysics and vibrational therapies. There was a time when I absolutely refused to contemplate anything that was defined by such words. I had a complete misunderstanding of what they meant and my mind was utterly closed to any further information about them.

One group of meanings given to the word esoteric according to the dictionary[1] is: something that is difficult to understand, abstruse, concealed or private.

These explanations seem to have been lost to its more common use in relation to an enlightened or initiated minority or restricted group, suggesting a cult or secret society. This latter meaning dominated my understanding of the word for many years. I use it in the context of something that is not

---

[1] Collins English Dictionary (Australian Edition), Updated Third Edition, HarperCollins Publishers, Sydney 1995.

obvious and when that something is discovered, it is not easy to understand.

The word metaphysics is equally misunderstood. Again, one of the meanings in the dictionary describe the word as a philosophical study of the nature of reality concerned with questions such as the existence of God and the external world. This explanation is the context in which I use the word: a philosophical study of the nature of the reality. In my case the reality is sickness and disease.

The more common meaning applied to this word is supernatural, which can conjure up thoughts of ghosts, poltergeist and mischievous spirits.

Albert Einstein gave the world the $E=mc^2$ equation, which simply means that energy and matter are interchangeable. Energy changes form into mass and vice versa. Therefore when I say I am interested in vibrational therapies, I am actually talking about Einstein's theory of change. Vibrational therapies change a particular vibration in the body. Vital life-giving energy has a different vibration to stagnant compressed energy which can change form in the body to a mass.

I still have a great love and passion for reflexology but my interest has moved from what it can do for someone to why that someone needed it in the first place.

Over the past ten or so years, I have investigated numerous complementary and alternative health modalities. The knowledge gained from these, plus the wisdom from my own personal and professional life experiences, has allowed me to consolidate what I have learnt and apply it within my own practice as something authentically my own. What I have come to believe has been confirmed by the response and feedback from many of my clients.

Encouraged by these results, I would like to share my findings with others.

The pages you are about to read explain reflexology from an holistic approach. I call my work *Holistic Reflexology*.

Supporting Beliefs

There are eight beliefs that are the forerunner to the work I do and why I do it. I did not always believe these things. Some of them I had never heard about until more recent years. Incorporating them into my belief system helped me to understand much of life that had previously made no sense because life was only ever considered through logic and the physical experience. They opened for me a bigger picture, a broader spectrum and a distant horizon that I had never considered before.

Your beliefs are not set in concrete. They can be readily changed. What you value, your ability to be open minded or your attachment to outcome, can be your catalyst to change, or your excuse to hold on to what doesn't serve you. There are many reasons to maintain a belief that you do not fully embrace: guilt, pleasing someone, being accepted or keeping the peace.

Beliefs that you hold on to that suppress your creative self-expressions and block your vital energy can be the underlying cause of your physical symptoms and undesirable life circumstances.

Belief # 1   Sickness will never be part of my life.

From the age of twenty-five until my early fifties, I would most probably have been described as a religious fanatic. In my mid-twenties I went searching for a deeper meaning to God, not unlike the search into the metaphysical realm in the past ten or so years.

One of the beliefs that attracted my attention when I was younger belonged to a somewhat controversial group within my church who were focused on healing. The more traditional thinkers promoted sickness as something sent from God to make a person stronger.

This posed a contradiction. If Jesus was going around healing everyone as the Bible told us and God had sent the illness in the first place to make a person stronger, Jesus got it wrong. I believed that Jesus got it right, which meant that sickness was not meant to be part of my life.

Jesus' contribution to the world didn't seem to be related to his health. It seemed to be more about compassion, empowerment and options. He moved outside the accepted parameters, challenged people's thinking and upset many in places of power and authority. I thought that would be a good model to follow.

In later years when I thought about it, sickness had been a big part of my life. My husband was diagnosed with type 1 diabetes over forty years ago which impacted, without question, on me and my family.

Belief # 2   Sore feet, disease and body symptoms are trying to draw my attention to something in my own life that needs to be addressed.

Feet issues and body symptoms are relatively easy to understand if you have the most basic knowledge of anatomy and physiology. The physical is reflecting the non-physical. If you understand the role of the physical, you can transpose it to what is not so obvious.

Your feet are not painful, tender and burning just to make your day unpleasant.

You don't have bunions simply to make your shopping experience for shoes difficult.

Sprained ankles aren't in support of the hot and cold pack industry.

Orthotics are not designed because of a bad shoe last.

Belief # 3   What I believe, I think about. What I think about with focus and emotion, I create.

I knew thoughts came from what I believed but for most of my life I had absolutely no idea that focusing on my thoughts produced a physical result or changed my life circumstances. I lived with the belief that God loved me and He would get me through anything that presented itself in my life.

Even though I hadn't heard about or realized that thought created, it still worked for me. Universal Law works whether you understand it or not, know about it or don't know about it, consciously put it into practice or use it in ignorance.

I have explained the relationship between thoughts and physical symptoms to my clients many times with the following story.

If you simply thought about a lion tearing you apart, you most probably wouldn't have any physical response. But what if you were in a situation where a lion actually walked up to you and stood a few metres away, snarling and watching you and there was nowhere for you to hide. Nowhere to run. No place to escape.

The lion hasn't done anything to you at this point but the thought of what is about to happen is now charged with emotion. Fear has combined with thought to create an automatic response in your body. It's more than likely that your bladder or bowel will release, your breathing change or your skin become pale and sweaty. And the lion hasn't even touched you. Your body is responding to thought.

As long as the lion remains unchallenged, your response may not change. Every effort to calm the effects the lion is having on you may be of no use.

If you tranquillize the lion and take it out of the scenario the cause has now been removed. Your bodily symptoms might well disappear quickly.

If fear can create such a strong bodily change in only a few minutes, then is it not possible that other emotions such as resentment, envy, hatred, anger or guilt could have a similar effect when attached to thoughts over a long period of time? Is it not possible that if you focus on these negative emotions over many years they too could create a physical change within your body?

A client once responded abruptly, "You're telling me it's all in my mind!" "No," I responded. "A tumour is real, broken bones are real, so are kidney stones and cancer. I am suggesting that what you think about plays a vital role in your health."

Belief # 4   To change my circumstances, I must change how I think about them.

Albert Einstein is quoted as saying, "You can't solve a problem with the same mind that created it." He obviously believed in the power of the mind to create.

Change your mind and you will change what you have created. Changing your beliefs can happen in an instant. Changing your thinking can take a little longer.

I have a lot more control over my mind than I used to have. It isn't allowed to go on and on like a cracked record. It is no longer able to control me with logic. I don't listen when it tells me what I should be doing, nor is it allowed to wallow in self-pity and victim-hood.

You can control what you think about. Nothing can stay in your mind unless you allow it to. It might take a little practice but the moment you become aware of any unwanted invasive thoughts, you can change them. Singing was one way I controlled my mind. It allowed me to change my focus to something else, similar to repeating a mantra.

I have embraced many changes in my life over the last fifteen years because I was able to recognize the beliefs I held on to and change how I thought about them, so that I could draw to myself circumstances of choice. Controlling my mind and changing my thinking was the beginning of the process.

Belief # 5   Energy cannot be created nor destroyed. It merely changes from one form to another.

As I became more interested in the metaphysical approach to life, I realized that science was at the forefront with explanations. When I thought about it, Albert Einstein's famous equation even supported my religious belief about life and death. My spirit is eternal and at death it simply changes form.

Science confirms that energy can neither be created nor destroyed, but merely changes from one form to another. The law of Conservation of Energy is one of the most fundamental and unbreakable laws of physics and is described in Einstein's famous equation $E=mc^2$. Energy and mass (matter) can change form back and forth.

When I thought about it, energy is energy, whether it is blocked or flowing freely. If energy can change form, then it was quite possible for suppressed, compacted or blocked energy to change form also. It became well within my scope of possibility that suppressed and blocked emotions could be compacted to form mass.

If awareness and information were being delivered to me in the form of energy and they were being ignored, then changing the delivery medium to mass could receive a better reception.

If emotions were ignored, maybe pain and symptoms wouldn't be.

Belief # 6   Chaos before Order.

I first heard about the Chaos before Order theory when I began to do Holosync Meditations.

I was confronted with a basic law of chemistry supporting a metaphysical concept. The further I moved into the metaphysical, the less proof I was searching for, while at the same time I was finding scientific evidence to support what I was discovering.

Ilya Prigogine was a Russian-born Belgian who worked in the field of physical chemistry. For his pioneering work in non-equilibrium thermodynamics, he was awarded The Nobel Prize in Chemistry in 1977. Prigogine proved his hypothesis that order emerges not in spite of chaos but because of it, that evolution and growth are the inevitable product of open systems slipping into temporary chaos and then reorganizing at higher levels of complexity. As humans, we are part of the open system.[2]

Therefore, *you must fall into temporary chaos* before reorganizing at a higher level of complexity. How long the temporary chaos lasts, is up to you.

Belief # 7   **I am responsible for everything in my life. On some level of my consciousness I have allowed, created or drawn to myself everything that is happening in my life.**

In the past, I might have said I was responsible for what was happening in my life, but somehow I didn't quite get the total concept of what responsibility was about.

Not only was I responsible for the more obvious decisions I had made, but I was also responsible on another level for absolutely everything that was a part of my life, even though I was not consciously aware of making a choice.

I chose many of my lessons before my birth and placed myself exactly into the most appropriate circumstances to achieve what I had set out to do. I believe that my life is far more extensive than my conscious memory can recall.

H'oponopono was the Kahuna belief that brought me a new awareness of the role I played in creating my own life circumstances, the role that others played in showing me myself and my issues, and a new understanding of God. While this awareness had been unfolding slowly, the H'oponopono Conference I attended in Hawaii consolidated all of that in a few days.

I am happy to accept responsibility for everything in my life because if I am the creator and I don't like what I see, then I can change it. It also means that no one has ever done anything to me. I have never been a victim.

It's easy to momentarily abdicate responsibility or fall into victim-hood, but the underlying beliefs I hold, quickly bring me back to a reality that is empowering and purposeful.

I create in one of two ways. I listen to divine inspiration and create from Source and Love, or I drag up old painful memories and belief patterns and recreate them over and over again.

---

[2] Bill Harris, Thresholds of the Mind, Centerpointe Research Institute, Inc. Washington, Oregon, 2002.

Belief # 8   I am God.

I attended the International Council of Reflexologists (ICR) Conference in Rome in 2001. It was one week after September 11 and the world was in chaos. Many people withdrew from the conference, including some of the speakers. Replacement presenters were found at short notice.

There was one speaker in particular, I can't remember the topic or her name, but she said five little words that were so far outside my boundaries and comfort zone that it would have been easier not to have heard them.

"You know you are God!"

She made that statement with such conviction that I felt I needed to take three steps backwards, even though I was sitting down, as the impact hit me. Then she looked at us all with somewhat disbelief that we may not have agreed with what she said.

It took me several years to process those words. My understanding of God has changed since I first heard them. What I believe about God and the universe now is very different to what I believed when I attended daily Mass for almost twenty-five years. While my beliefs have changed, I am grateful for the foundations upon which they were built.

I believe that the relative universe is God in experience. As nothing can exist outside of God or Source, the apparent separation we feel is the illusion necessary to allow the experience. That, I believe, is what we are here to understand and experience.

This final belief underpins and overrides everything else I consider or accept. It is my empowerment, the reason I am here and the explanation for everything that logic denies.

Introduction

The body is programmed to heal itself. Cells are intelligent, have memory and communicate with each other. If I cut my finger the healing process begins immediately, and before long new skin appears.

Over the years, I have torn several patches of skin off my arm. My arm is now healed, but I have been left with scars. If scarring is part of the healing process and my arm has healed and skin is replaced every month or so, why do I still have scars on my arm many years after the event? What happened to change the memory of the cells so that they reproduced in the scarring pattern, not the original skin pattern?

Those thoughts led me to ask the question, "When something else in the body needs healing and healing isn't happening, what is negating the healing process?" Has the cellular memory been changed as well? Are the cells holding on to some trauma which is affecting how they function and communicate with each other?

Feet hold the answers to many unresolved questions about health and life in general.
- Sore feet are not trying to make life unpleasant.
- Sore feet are trying to give you a message.
- Sore feet are trying to draw attention to what area of life needs to be addressed.

While traditional reflexology would suggest that the whole body is mapped on the feet, I believe that the whole person is seen there as well. Not only are the parts of the body identifiable on the feet, but everything that contributes to the totality of the person is also represented. By considering the metaphysical connection between the foot, body and lifestyle, it can be easier than you might think to discover a starting point to what is blocking the healing process.

The fact that I will introduce a client to a possibility doesn't necessarily mean they will follow the idea through, nor does it mean that the foot pain will disappear. Many clients simply have sore feet, nothing more, nothing less. Many other clients have symptoms unrelated to lifestyle and choices, and diseases which they have inherited through no choice of their own.

In my practice I apply eight principles, which collectively I have called *Holistic Reflexology*.

#1 Anatomy and physiology reflect another perspective
#2 Chakras reveal flow and blockages in energy
#3 Elements express their energy through the toes
#4 Organs hold emotions, often suppressed
#5 Left and right define who, how and when
#6 Shape, texture and position show strength and weakness, potential and challenge
#7 Words and phrases draw a parallel to the cause
#8 I attract my own issues

Following these principles will, most times, give me a starting point. Some clients will instantly understand the connection, others may take a little while, and others will never see the relevance.

The natural progression of evolution pushes us ever forward to consciousness. Whether or not we co-operate with this process defines the sort of life experiences we will create. How one describes such experiences depends on one's perspective on life in general. If we pay attention and allow this vital energy to flow and create, then it is possible that good health will embrace us.

If you make choices which stagnate and block this vital life force, then it is possible that your energy will become compacted and cause damage to your health, wellbeing and lifestyle.

Feet tell the story of the body
The body speaks for the soul
All too often
Logic takes control
The mind interprets
Intuition is ignored
The messages of the feet are lost to physical pain
and
Potential for growth passes by unnoticed

15

Holistic Reflexology Principle # 1
Anatomy and physiology reflect another perspective

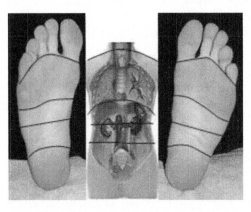

This principle is not intended to be another anatomy and physiology manual. There are many excellent books already available on the subject. I am presuming that the reader has an understanding of the various parts of the body, their overall role and how they work. Nor is this book intended to be a reflexology manual. Once again, there are excellent books written about the practical application of reflexology. However, I have included, at the end of the book, the reflexes which I use in my reflexology practice.

Principle #1 invites you to expand your basic knowledge of anatomy and physiology, look at the body systems from a metaphysical perspective, and discover the connection your pain and symptoms have to your daily life.

Like other forms of esoteric communication, it comes in concepts, symbols and possibilities. So in trying to interpret what the body is saying, you may need to listen with a conceptual approach rather than a logical one.

Isolating the components of a body system identifies the role each one plays, and how it individually contributes to the overall success of that system when everything is functioning unimpeded.

One of the keys to understanding what the body is trying to communicate through your feet is knowing:
- how your body works
- what function each organ performs
- what your body systems do for you

It is relatively straightforward to translate the physical to the metaphysical if you know what role the source of discomfort or disease plays in your body.

- Nervous System is about communication and interpreting
- Endocrine System focuses on authority figures and learning through negative feedback
- Cardiovascular System is connected to flow and blockages and being on the right track
- Lymphatic System and Immunity is associated with picking up after others, self-protection and self-criticism
- Skeletal System gives structure, restructure and infrastructure
- Muscular System is about divided loyalties as it pulls in two directions
- Digestive System has a lot to do with process and teamwork as it assimilates and disposes
- Respiratory System deals with fair exchange and transition
- Urinary System is about monitoring, balance and recycling
- Reproductive System develops creative expression
- Integumentary System defines boundaries, security and a willingness to be on show
- Special Senses give you a way to remember

In the pages ahead I will provide an overview of the body systems from a metaphysical perspective, that is, a philosophical study of the nature of the reality of sickness and disease, with the hope of bringing forth in the reader an abstract discussion within themselves.

Nervous System

I control your communication
I connect your outside world to your inside world
I interpret your experiences and prepare you for your reply

Overview

The nervous system is the body's major form of communication. Any discomfort and dysfunction associated with it is related in some way to your ability to communicate with others. When part of the nervous system is under stress, it is more than likely that some form of your personal communication is under stress as well.

You may think you are collecting information with an open mind when in reality you have an agenda to which you do not admit, emotions that overrule you and behaviour patterns that you have not yet consciously recognized. Any of these underlying issues can impinge on the way you collect your information, inhibit your ability to process without bias, and affect the end result. You either, don't get the message as was intended, or the recipient has no idea what you are trying to communicate.

People can't read your mind, so don't presume that they can. Say what you mean, be straightforward in presenting your needs, and ask questions if you don't understand. Most importantly, don't expect others to analyze something in the same way that you do.

All of the frustrations and disruptions in your personal communication add to a breakdown in the nervous system.

Metaphysics of the Nervous System

Central Nervous System
   Brain
      Unlimited potential and much of it unused
      Who is in control?

Spinal Cord

Working closely with someone can be quite difficult and challenging
Take care that the appropriate person receives the correct information
You need to pass on the information accurately whether you approve or not
You may be misinterpreting

Peripheral Nervous System

I am delicate
I damage easily
I need to be protected
I need others around me to give me strength
I do not function on my own

Autonomic Nervous System

I have no control over what is happening
I am unable to make any change
I am a victim

Somatic Reflexes

I will make this work for me if it's the last thing I do

Messages of the Nervous System

Communication is but a way
For two hearts to unite in understanding
On a level that brings
Growth, love and evolvement

Identify any prejudices you have which affect how you listen, understand and communicate.

Your communication skills may need to be improved to take into consideration how the other person listens.

Disagreements can cause problems resulting in a breakdown in communications. Try to see the situation from the other person's perspective.

You may have a need to talk to someone you are estranged from but they may not want to talk to you.

A closed mind and fixed ideas can reject anything that is not compatible with them.

Words have different meanings for different people, and your message may not be understood as you intended it to be.

Information can be collected and distributed in different ways. Some forms of communication are conceptual while others are specific.

Once the information has been gathered, it can be distorted as you process it through your own value and belief system.

Examples

- Female client presented with Morton's neuroma on the right foot which had been treated with a cortisone injection, giving relief for about three weeks. The client and her husband had been travelling in Australia for several years and had spent the past twelve months working in a very remote area. This was when the problem began. I asked how she kept in touch with her family while she was away. She used email and phone and believed that was satisfactory.

  Hugging someone with feeling is different to holding a phone and sending words. Emails don't come close to sitting down for a coffee and chat. When someone persists in wanting to know when you are coming home, the existing forms of communication would appear not to be satisfactory. A close family member developed a Morton's neuroma simultaneously with the client.

- A young woman came to see if reflexology could help Parkinson's disease. Her condition had developed to the point where she needed support to walk. All of her family, except her partner, lived in another country. She was chronically homesick, had no close friends and felt cut off from almost everyone she loved. Her communication network didn't exist.

Endocrine System

I monitor your performance
Negative feedback is my measuring stick
My leader tells you when you need to give more
Constructive comment is different from personal criticism

Overview

The endocrine system is also a communication network. It has an authority figure that keeps a close eye on the other organs in the group, and networks through chemical messages.

The leader is acutely sensitive to the levels needed to function at optimum efficiency and is able to pick up what needs to be done by identifying what is not present. The success of this system is based on negative feedback because the organ in charge has an overall view, whereas each individual member is more focused on itself.

The leader encourages the others in the group to listen, and respond when asked. The leader doesn't do the work of producing the hormones and enzymes, but expects the others in the system to do it themselves under direction.

When any part of this system is in distress, constructive comment may have been misinterpreted for personal criticism. Someone's innate creative skills could have been thwarted, or a member of the team could be negating their responsibilities and adding to the workload of others.

A breakdown in this system could also indicate a person has issues with their boss or authority figures in general.

If you refuse to listen and respond to your spiritual inner guidance, you may also find discomfort in these areas of your body.

Metaphysics of the Endocrine System

Pituitary and Hypothalamus
    Supporting the spiritual, mental, physical and emotional growth of others
    Listening and co-operating with others
    Helping others with their creative pursuits
    Sabotaging the natural flow of events

Pineal
    Blocking the Light
    Refusing to shed light on an issue
    Refusing to see options
    Closed mind

Thyroid
    Burning yourself out
    Imbalance
    Giving too much of yourself
    Not pulling your weight

Parathyroid
    Breaking down structures
    Redirection
    Locked into a position

Thymus
    Self-protection
    Keeping the enemy at bay
    Bravery
    Assertiveness
    Bolstering yourself up to do something

Adrenals
    You are under stress
    Do you fight for, flee from or freeze?
    Expecting the worst to happen

Pancreas
    The ability to take what you have and what you have learned, and make it work for you
    Not using the resources on hand
    Not able to make use of your resources in a positive way
    Unable to tap into your resources
    Support coming to me from higher up the chain may be blocked

Gonads
See Reproductive System

Messages of the Endocrine System

The orchestra is led by the master conductor
No instrument plays until it is directed
Everyone has their own arrangement
Each is gifted and creative
Together they perform a masterpiece

Constructive comment is fruitful when it is not misinterpreted as personal criticism.

Listening for what is not said and what is not done can be more informative than what is.

There are situations where someone needs to be in control. If you have a problem with authority figures in general, you may not appreciate good leadership.

Some people have a tendency to take over and do everything rather than delegate, and allow others to do things in their own way.

Learning to balance what you give to others with what you need for yourself will save you from burnout.

You need to learn when to say, "No."

You can only put on a brave face for a certain length of time. Appearances are eventually seen through.

Be grateful for the gifts and abilities you have, and put them to work for you. They will grow and develop as you use them.

Integrate what you learn into your life.

When you stop and face your problems, you may find they cease to pursue you.

Define your stress and break it down into workable pieces.

Examples

- A client came to see me because his feet had been very sore for about two months. He began wearing new shoes about two months before, and surprisingly enough had started a new job about two months ago as well. He thought the shoes were the problem. I asked him if he liked the new job. "It's a job," he replied, which immediately told me he didn't particularly like it.

  He didn't say much at all during the first session, and as he was leaving, told me that he had just gone onto medication. He obviously didn't think it was related to his sore feet, or he would have mentioned it earlier. The medication was for type 2 diabetes. His efforts to maintain control by diet had failed, and he felt deeply disappointed by having to yield to medication.

  When he came back the following week, I suggested that diabetes could be related to one of two things. Because it is an immune system disease, he might consider if he was being overly self-critical or, because the pancreas is part of the endocrine system, were there any situations where he was learning through negative feedback. He needed to ask himself if he was criticizing himself unduly, or if someone was trying to teach him something that he was taking as personal criticism.

  This client had changed careers several times and appeared to be able to put his hand to anything but this new job was in a field that he had avoided for most of his life.

  I asked him how he got on with his boss, to which he replied, "He's never satisfied."

  I suggested that the boss could be trying to help him learn, and he was taking it personally; only hearing criticism. Also what he considered to be negative feedback could actually be a positive, to help him learn and improve. He only came a few times and his feet were noticeably better.

- A lady presented with plantar fasciitis (pulled in two directions) around the sacral chakra area (power games) of the right foot. Her adrenal reflexes were stressed on the right foot, which drew my foremost attention.

  She was on holidays, walking on the beach when her foot became sore. I asked what she was thinking about at the time. She told me how much she loved the place. Her holiday was almost finished, and she was about to go home. Her adult son had recently come back home to live. She was pulled in two directions. She loved him, but she didn't want him living with her. Throughout the whole treatment she kept a close eye on the time as she needed to be home by 7.00 pm to cook dinner for him. I did ask why he couldn't cook it for himself.

The metaphysics of the adrenals in relation to the endocrine system is about doing things for yourself, not having others do them for you. I really enjoyed the chat we had but she didn't come back for a second session.

Cardiovascular System

I deliver your needs and remove some debris
My heart gives you the reason, love
My vessels give you the pathway, trust
My blood gives you the passion, fullness of life

Overview

The cardiovascular system is the major transport system of the body. Discomfort associated with this area is related to flow or stagnation in your life. This system will function to the degree that love flows through your life, and your needs are met. When love, trust and passion are blocked, and you become stagnant, the system will collapse or simply give up.

The heart is the symbol of love, and love is the never-ending energy to guide you along the pathways that lead to fulfilment and happiness. You may try to bypass love, but love is an innate need of the human soul, and love will have its place. Side stepping is but a temporary measure; one day it will hold you accountable.

Your blood vessels symbolize an intricate pathway for you to follow, your road map guiding you in the right direction. When your journey is rough, you may reach a place that feels comfortable. So, you create for yourself road blocks to keep you there for a little while, to allow you to regroup and consider the options. Pain and discomfort can follow you as you try to escape the pathway. It's like swimming against the flow, or wading upstream against the current. It is exhausting trying to avoid what you must face up to in life.

If blood is your passion, then here you will find the yardstick for how you engage life. Life is a process of cycles. The secret is to use the wisdom of your heart to know: when each cycle is complete, when the next will begin, and what to take with you or leave behind.

Metaphysics of the Cardiovascular System

Heart
>Your ability to love
>Love never tires, ends or counts the cost
>Working for the good of the whole

Vessels
>The path to follow
>Going with the flow

Blood
>**White Blood cells**
>>Under attack
>>Expecting a battle at any moment
>>Your defences are up

>**Red Blood cells**
>>Body cycles
>>The importance of recognizing the use-by date
>>Taking it with you or leaving it behind

>**Platelets**
>>Sticking together
>>Ganging up
>>Closed ranks
>>The initial response

Messages of the Cardiovascular System

I am the stream that flows gently to the river
The river that flows freely to the ocean
The ocean that carries you to the furthest horizon
Always arriving at your perfect destination

Love with conditions is not love. It is a quantified response to a given situation. Unconditional love holds no agenda, no expectations, no judgments. It is far removed from the conscious nature of humans, and yet at the same time, is their intrinsic spiritual essence.

Unconscious beliefs that rule your life can convince you that you are constantly under attack.

Being on guard, ready for the battle, puts your army in a different position. Instead of wearing red to draw forth your passion and excitement, they wear white with the expectation that their life force will be drained and exhausted.

If you are not able to give up what is fatigued and of no further use to you, your life journey becomes slow and tedious, and your potential under-utilized.

The wisdom of your heart will tell you when something has reached its use-by date. You might need to consider why you continue to hold on to people and patterns that do not serve your highest good.

There is a difference between living your life with passion, and existing in circumstances perceived to be outside of your control. You have the ability to change what it is that steals your passion.

As you move through the cycles of your life, remember what you have learnt. Take it with you, and apply it to your future.

Sticking together to achieve something is one thing. Becoming an exclusive group is another.

There are some things that can't be done as an individual. Know when you need the support of others. Be ready to give acknowledgment when it is due.

The initial response is sometimes more of a reaction. Your initial response to something may be inappropriate, and your first impressions of someone may need to be reassessed.

There is a difference between going with the flow in a group, and flowing with the intuition of your heart. Flowing with the group may give an appearance of peace while turmoil rules beneath. Intuitive following may initially appear chaotic, but the underpinning wisdom will eventually bring calmness and stability.

Example

- When I left school, my first job was in an office. The manager of the business eventually became one of the first people in Australia to have a heart transplant. I find it interesting that just a few years after someone receives a new heart, they can die from the same disease that destroyed the first one.

28

Lymphatic System and Immunity

I am the defence force
I supply the army to do battle with the enemy
I stand at attention waiting to be called into action

Overview

The lymphatic system is one of the major transport systems, on call for your defence. Its main concern is cleaning up the debris and keeping your body clear of waste. Its army is on standby to attack and defeat the enemy at any given moment, restoring peace and harmony. Discomfort and symptoms appearing in this system are drawing your attention to your tendency to pick up after others, putting your physical and emotional wellbeing at risk in the meantime.

Your lymph is ceaselessly picking up what another part of the body has left on the roadside as waste. No sooner does the lymph pick up the mess, sweep and tidy, dust and polish than it is time to go back and do it all again. When picking up after others never seems to come to an end, it becomes despairing, but it's the negative emotions of others that you pick up that drain you even more.

Co-dependence and lymph are closely related. When the volatile residue of another is left for you to absorb or dispose of, and your moment by moment state of mind depends on how that person is acting towards you, your co-dependence may show up in this system.

Living in fear and apprehension of the next battle will stress your spleen. It builds and holds its resources just in case. When you are expecting to be attacked at any moment and are on alert for the next battle, it is more than likely that a problem will arise in this system. The mentality of *What if* and *Just in case* sit close by.

The early baby boomer years brought with them an epidemic of tonsillectomies. Children in that era weren't allowed to speak up. Can you imagine how many words must have been kept in and swallowed? How much self-expression suppressed? Children didn't put on tantrums like today.

Children did as they were told; in those years, children conformed. All that anger didn't come out, and it didn't go down either. It just sat in the throat and fermented. The poor tonsils! When they became inflamed and angry, they were removed. Was it wishful thinking that outspoken, provocative children could simply be removed?

The immune response is more focused on self-protection. It has the ability to recognize the enemy, and send out the special forces to do battle. It remembers all previous encounters, and mounts a stronger response each time the enemy attacks. Revenge remembers everything, and makes sure the enemy is held accountable. Revenge contributes to the breakdown in immunity.

Overreacting to something is also an immune issue, and it shows up in your allergies and hay fever, as the body overreacts in its response to a given situation.

Metaphysics of the Lymphatic System and Immunity

Lymph
 Dumping on someone
 Picking up after others
 Knowing your boundaries

Spleen
 Expecting the next emergency
 On stand-by
 Ready for battle
 Expecting to be attacked
 Keeping your guard up
 Defence strategy collapsing
 Support removed

Thymus
 Focused learning
 Education

Tonsils
 Taking it all in to be sorted out later
 Having something rammed down your throat
 Having to swallow/accept things that are foreign to you
 Angry words being contained

Peyer's Patches
>Hidden, subtle ways to use against others
>Ready for attack

Immune Response
>The enemy will be eliminated
>I will never forget what you did to me
>There is no hiding place
>Anger
>Revenge
>Overreacting

Messages of the Lymphatic System and Immunity

I am the street cleaner who comes out after dark
I work almost unnoticed to pick up after the day's busy events
I collect what is no longer wanted
That which has been discarded by the roadside
Left there for someone else to attend to

Your state of calm and your peace of mind do not depend on whether someone else is having a good or bad day. It depends on you.

When you continue to pick up after others, are you really helping them, or satisfying a need within yourself.

The problem with picking up the emotions of another is that you might begin to think they are yours. They are reflecting something about you, but they don't belong to you.

What are the things that you are capable of doing for yourself that you choose not to do, resulting in someone else having to do them for you?

If you believe in universal guidance, there is no such thing as the next emergency.

When you criticize and attack yourself, your personal army may mistake who the enemy is, and attack you instead of protecting you. Be kind to yourself.

When you are expecting the worst and you are feeling vulnerable, attack seems your best line of defence. Where did you learn that everyone is out to get you?

31

Keeping track of every move the enemy makes and matching every manoeuvre might have benefits if you were really at war, but if it's only to help plan revenge, then the attack is more aimed at yourself.

If you can't be grateful for what someone has done to you, then accept it. If you can't accept it, seek forgiveness. Ask them to forgive you, because on some level of your consciousness, you have forgotten that you gave your permission.

Sometimes you just need to get over your overreaction.

Have you ever entered into something with good intentions and somehow ended up 'the bad guy'? That is when you have to remember why you got involved in the first place. Don't mistake the real enemy.

It's one thing to be aware of what needs attention in your life. It's another thing to do something about it. Do you know what needs to be cleaned up? When are you going to address it?

Examples

- While working with someone's feet one day, my mind was still, and I began to drift. I found myself in an old fashioned country kitchen.

  There was a short, stocky lady in a white apron tending to a large metal pot on a big wood stove. There was a long wooden table in the centre of the room. When the meal was ready, she called for everyone to come and eat, but no one came. She waited and waited, and then became very angry, so decided to throw the meal out, but when she took the lid off the pot, she saw that she had been boiling the washing not cooking a meal. While she thought she was cooking the meal and nurturing them, she was actually doing their washing and picking up after them.

  The message of the story was: We need to learn how much is enough when it comes to what we do for family, friends and business associates. If we have become a slave to their needs, we need to look at what motivates us. Sometimes we get confused. We need to be able to tell the difference between supporting bad habits, and nurturing, loving and caring.

  Maybe somewhere years ago "it" became your job, and even though circumstances have changed, the dynamics haven't. Maybe it's time to renegotiate certain things. Maybe you continue to clean up after others because it's easier than confrontation. It's time to put things in their right place.

- When young adults suffer with tonsillitis I have to wonder if what is being thrust down their necks is foreign to everything they deem important.

Skeletal System

I am your infrastructure
I connect you with others
I am flexible, yet fixed at the same time

Overview

Discomfort associated with the skeletal system is related to the degree of support you feel from others, how you stand in relationship to them, and how you connect with them or protect yourself from them. It will draw your attention to what is being restructured, the effectiveness of your support network, and how safe you feel in the world at large.

Just imagine if your bones were not connected to each other, you would merely be an unrecognizable heap on the floor. How you connect to others tells you much about yourself. How you connect to others helps you recognize yourself, and define the issues you need to deal with in your own life. Your relationships are your mirror image. You need to move through any emotional reaction before you will be able to see your own reflection.

The skeletal system is your physical infrastructure, the support system you have set up to project and maintain your life choices. As your beliefs are the ultimate infrastructure that project and maintain your life choices, you may find problems with this body system when your beliefs need to be reassessed because the protocols in place no longer support what you believe or who you have become.

Just as your bones give you form, strength and structure, your real strength is within, not without. Your character, developed by endurance and perseverance creates your integrity. Your integrity, while not seen, is always noticed.

Metaphysics of the Skeletal System

Bone
> Infrastructure
> Restructuring
> Protection
> Inner strength
> Storage

Connective Tissue
> **Cartilage**
> Temporary support
> Growing into your own strength
> Definition

> **Dense Connective Tissue**
> **Ligaments and Tendons**
> Connecting to and disconnecting from others
> Tied to or torn apart
> Wearing thin
> Holding on

> **Loose Connective Tissue**
> **Areola**
> Keeping everything in place
> Order
> **Adipose**
> Protection and cushioning

Joints
> Approach to life
> Ability to relate

Messages of the Skeletal System

I am the infrastructure, the unseen, the invisible
I give form, shape and appearance
I am the foundation, your strength within
That is what makes you stand apart and be noticed...
The unseen strength within

Your infrastructure may be fine and delicate yet incredibly strong. Appearances can be deceiving.

If you continually say that you need a break from what you are doing, you may well break a bone. Choose your words carefully as they are the foundation of what you create.

Bones draw on their own inner strength. From where do you draw yours?

Some forms of support are only meant to be temporary. Recognize when your temporary support has served its purpose. Let it go, and grow in your own strength. Scaffolding surrounds a building only until it can stand alone. Then it is taken down.

When you choose to rely on others for support when you are able to do it for yourself, you may find your cartilage will deliver a message about your own abilities.

Learn to recognize the difference between what appears to be temporary, but is actually long term, and what is temporary, in transition.

Tearing or breaking connective tissue can be an indication to let go of controlling others, or a need to break away from the control others have over you.

You may be tied to another so closely that you are losing your self-identity.

You may have disconnected from someone, and you have a sense of being torn apart.

Fat tissue can suggest issues relating to perfection and control. You may have a place for everything and everybody in your life, and everything and everybody must stay in their proper place. You may be black and white in your outlook on life.

Alternatively, your life may be in such chaos and disorder that no one knows where they stand. No one knows their place.

Fat tissue could be telling you that you do not readily allow others to bring you warmth, so you have to provide that for yourself.

When you are overly protected by your own fat tissue, you need to discover who or what you are insulating yourself against.

Lack of fat tissue could be saying that you feel you do not deserve to be kept warm, protected and insulated.

Look to your joints to discover how flexible or fixed your relationships are. Relationships are not all meant to work the same, nor are they all compatible. Some will only go in one direction, others will be limited and restricted, while some will move freely. When a relationship is under stress, your joints can give you an idea of what needs correction or attention.

Examples

- A middle aged man presented with a right foot problem. He had fractured the same bone three times over the last two years. He thought reflexology might help to strengthen the foot. I wondered if anything in his life had been restructured. After some quiet time, he told me that his wife had been diagnosed with cancer. The whole family dynamics had changed. The infrastructure of the family came under threat.

- A client was overworked and exhausted. She kept thinking to herself, "I need a break." She broke her collar bone. She told me after the event that she should have had more sense than to use such a term. She needed to restructure her life and create a balance between work and family. Pity she had to break a bone before she took notice.

- A young woman in her early twenties presented with left shoulder pain. The doctors told her it was related to tendons. I was eager to learn when the problem began, and what she was doing at the time. I suggested that tendons are connective tissue and that the underlying cause may be related to how she connected with others.
  "Could it be about disconnecting from others?" she asked.
  She had only recently returned from working with women in a third world country. The pain began as soon as she arrived home. She had become very close to these women during her stay with them. Disconnecting from them was emotionally painful for her. She felt she was leaving part of her family behind.
  I believe that acknowledging the emotion attached to a particular situation is all that is sometimes needed to dissipate the pain. Sometimes the body will heal. Sometimes it won't. There are many multi-level issues being dealt with at the same time.

- I've met several middle aged men facing redundancy. They all had a right hip problem. One of the things that the right hip is related to is material security and power games. It wasn't surprising that these men, who were concerned with employment, money and stability, had something showing in that area of their body. They were all faced with restructuring their physical work and finances.

- A woman client had problems with her legs, ankles and feet since she was a child. Her main concern was her right lower leg. She had suffered with osteomyelitis as a child, and the leg had been a problem to her for most of her life. She also told me a little about her mother. During the Second World War when my client was a child, her father received a call-up to the army. Her mother said that if he joined she would leave him, which she did. In the following years the child would be belted if she was polite to the father when he came to visit. Eventually he stopped coming.

  The child's life had changed dramatically when the family had broken up, and it wasn't all that long until the bone infection began. The leg settled down for many years until my client's marriage broke up, when once again she found herself restructuring her life.

Muscular System

I give you the ability to move freely and participate in life
I help you create your choices
I am here to give you the experience
Choose wisely

Overview

The muscular system is associated with growth through a physical experience. New experiences extend your horizon, open your mind and present possibility. All of us are invited to take part in these new adventures, but only the brave will explore them and reap the benefits of the experience.

Discomfort associated with the muscular system is related to the choices you are making in your life. If you are suffering pain or trauma through your muscles, you may have to look at the decisions you make, why you make them and whether change is appropriate.

Some muscles work automatically, others on command. You may find that some of your actions are no longer conscious choices for they have become automatic, habitual and repetitive. Muscle pain is often connected to pressure and expectation of others, rather than conscious choices made for your own greater good.

Muscles work in pairs, one pulls and the other pushes. Muscle pain can be related to being pulled in two directions, divided loyalties and not knowing which way to go.

You may also need to isolate the degree of pain your muscles hold because you do not live up to the expectations and pressures others put upon you. When you insist on incessantly working for others and do not consider your own needs, muscles can become so fatigued they refuse to work for anybody. Guilt is a driving force that will never give you rest.

Trying to live up to what others expect from you will exhaust you. Living your life according to what you should be doing is existing, not living. It can be a positive experience to use your muscles and energy for others, but it's the intention that goes with the action that will drain or invigorate you. You will know your intention by the response in your body.

Use your energy well. Keep your muscles happy. Learn to balance your actions. Let your choices honour yourself. You are not selfish.

Metaphysics of the Muscular System

Skeletal Muscles
Shoulder, neck and face
Carrying the load
Looking in another direction

Diaphragm
Relaxation
Breath of life

Lower trunk
Core strength
A pain in the butt

Arm
Reaching out
Flexing my muscle
Giving and receiving

Leg
Stepping out
Taking risks
Following the leader
Changing direction
In a hurry

Smooth muscle of organs
Automatic responses
Habitual behaviour
Lost control

Cardiac muscle
Lifetime commitments
Time out

Messages of the Muscular System

I give you a blank canvas. What will you create?
Black and white... dull and dreary
Vibrant colours... cheerful and bright
You hold the brush
You decide. It's your choice
Are you ready to create your own masterpiece

When the load is heavier than you imagined it would be, give yourself permission to put it down. Maybe it belongs to someone else anyway.

The weight of carrying responsibility for others can be overwhelmingly painful. Strength of character is not measured by your muscles.

While you stay focused on what is before you, know what is in your peripheral sights. Look around, distract your tunnel vision, keep up with what's happening.

The best choice you might ever make is to take a few deep breaths while you reassess what is going on, and what your response will be.

The power games you play will resonate in your muscles as you pull and push at each other. Your core energy will be drained and redirected as you argue and fight for the dominant position. What price are you prepared to pay?

In your reaching out to give, be sure you are able to hold your hands out to receive.

If you decide to flex your muscles and address a particular issue, make sure you have collected all the relevant information beforehand. When you stand up to be counted, you will often find you are on your own.

Give yourself permission to change direction, or go back and begin again. Back tracking isn't about failure. When you discover new information and know that it will benefit you, it takes wisdom to recognize the fact, and courage to act.

Sometimes you will need another to walk with you along your life path, other times you won't. Sometimes you will be the leader, other times you will follow. It doesn't matter if others don't understand, nor does it matter if others don't give their permission. This is your life path to walk, etched by your choices.

41

Give the knowing of your heart permission to lead you. Recognize when your automatic reactions surface to protect and defend you, your logic dominates, and your emotions control you. Notice the areas of your life where you feel you have no control.

Give yourself permission to reassess a long term commitment. Allow yourself to change your mind. Others may not give you permission to change your choices. You may have to give it to yourself.

Examples

- An elderly lady had suffered with restless leg syndrome for many years. It was particularly bad in the evening when she sat down. She usually kept two televisions on, so she could sit down for a little while in the lounge and stand up in another room. This was how she watched television until her legs settled, and she could sit down and relax again. She wasn't particularly open to the way I thought. Eventually, she told me that every time she sat down as a child her father would hit her over the head with a rolled up newspaper, and tell her not to be lazy.

  She was still being pulled in two directions. The needs of the adult were opposing the response of the child. She had never addressed the issue of her father, so it still dominated part of her life.

- A woman came with lower back problems on the left side in the sacral and base chakra areas, which made me think about her place in the family and power games. She had also suffered with plantar fasciitis for the past eighteen months. She was estranged from one of her sisters, with no sign of reconciliation. She was being pulled in two directions and didn't know what the next move would be.

- A client presented with sore feet. I began by asking about her general state of health. She was able to list off many conditions and symptoms, but then stopped. She wanted to know what that had to do with having a foot massage. I explained the principle of reflexology and that she couldn't have her feet done without having some response in other parts of her body.

  I began working very lightly, which is not my usual style. She couldn't seem to settle. I felt she was edgy the whole time, just waiting in expectation for the next part to hurt. I would guess that is how she lived her life, waiting for the next thing to happen.

  Her feet reminded me of someone being trapped in a cage, but it wasn't something I continued to explore. There are times when I

42

know it is better not to continue with my line of thought or conversation. Some people just have sore feet.

- A client presented with fibromyalgia and very low energy levels. One of her children had ongoing difficulties within the marriage and she knew that if she intervened, the effects would flow on to her grandchildren. Her heart was pulling her one way, while her logic and reasoning the other. She was being pulled in two directions from within.

Digestive System

I take it in
I churn it around
I use what is beneficial and dispose of the rest
Chaos before order

Overview

The digestive system is about process, discernment and teamwork; knowing what is of benefit to you and what is not. It has the ability to transform the solids you eat into the chemicals that will nourish and sustain your cells. It is wise enough to know what to dispose of, but you can sabotage the process by clinging on to what is no longer of any use.

Your body is a combination of complex chemicals that work together to attain an end result. This system has lessons about working with others through a process. Each component is required to do the best they can. Each part of the process depends on the previous work done. If one part isn't working, then there is a good chance it will affect what will happen next.

Many people find that their digestive system is no longer able to process wheat and dairy, two of the most staple foods in our society. When this system is under stress, it is possible that there are issues relating to nurturing in the physical sense resulting in a lack of stability.

Stability is linked to process. If you move from one thing to another before you have been able to process and integrate the information or experience, then the end result may be instability. If as a child you experienced many changes, and were not able to process one before the next began, digestive issues may well present themselves later in life.

Metaphysics of the Digestive System

Alimentary Canal
Mouth and tongue
> Touching the senses
> Clarity

Pharynx
> Common passage way
> Confined space shared with someone else

Esophagus
> Something to swallow
> Pathway to follow

Stomach
> Turning upside down
> Uncertainty
> Process in place
> Taking time

Small Intestine
> Using your resources
> Appropriate use
> Discerning what benefits you
> Absorption

Illeocecal Valve
> Living in the past
> Closing off from the past
> Moving forward

Appendix
> Nowhere to go
> Dead end
> Up against a brick wall

Large Intestine
> Refusing to let go of the past
> Hanging on
> Compacting old hurts
> Moving through a process too quickly
> Needing to slow down and let others do their job
> What else can you glean from a given situation?

Sigmoid colon
>Change of direction
>A need to keep moving

Rectum
>Letting go
>Strain and effort
>Relief

Accessory Digestive Organs
Teeth
>Biting off more than you can chew
>Rocking your foundations
>Breaking things down

Saliva Glands
>Doing things the hard way
>I can make this easier

Pancreas
>Neutralize the situation

Gall Bladder
>Dissolving your protection
>Neutralizing a situation

Liver
>Detoxify all levels
>Ability to allocate
>Balance of masculine and feminine
>Regenerate, re-grow
>Storage
>Monitoring the situation
>Supply and demand

Messages of the Digestive System

I am the trash and treasure, the garage sale, the market stand
I accept it all, sort it out
Put to work what is useful
Get rid of the junk
And start the process all over again

Some things in life are sweet, others are bitter. Some you will swallow readily, others you will spit out. There are some lessons that must be taken. Taste is irrelevant.

Being put in a position where you have to work with people you don't like can bring out the worst in you, but it can also bring out the best, if you can see them as a teacher reflecting your issues back to you. Here lies a golden opportunity for self-development.

The difficult things in life are easier to accept when you look for the positives. They may not be obvious, but they are there. You find what you focus on.

Life will often fall into chaos while it is in the process of finding a new order. How long the chaos lasts depends on your perception of what is happening.

Some things in life simply need time. They can't be hurried, coerced or manipulated. They just need a little time. Some lessons appear infuriatingly slow. Some people just need a little patience and tolerance.

Uncertainty is a definite. There are no guarantees that you will get what you hope for, but whatever happens, you can use it to your advantage.

Be grateful for who and what you are. Develop and apply your resourcefulness. Put what you have learnt into practice, and let it work for you. Stop wishing you were someone else.

Nothing will ever match the memory of the past, not even the past itself.

There is no such place as a dead end or brick wall, just detours and redirection. Some roads are impassable, and because you had to take the detour, you are never going to see what you have missed.

You need to make space to let the new enter, but the real benefit is that when there is space and the new comes, you can choose where to put it.

Toxic waste is just as real in your body as in the environment. Give your body some time to process what it lets go of, and avoid a healing crisis. Too much too soon can have repercussions.

There's always more than one way to do something, and sometimes the best way is another person's idea.

Examples

- A client was in the process of setting up a business in partnership with others. It had almost reached the point of no return when the stock market took a major correction. It was as though all the hard work and planning might come to nothing. Had the project reached a brick wall with nowhere to go? He had an emergency operation to remove his appendix.

- A young mother was concerned about her eight year old daughter. She was chronically constipated. I asked the woman about the relationship with her husband. They had separated. She was very bitter. She told me she couldn't let go. The daughter was holding the mother's emotion in her bowel. The woman needed to deal with her own relationship issues before the daughter would improve.

- A young woman came to see me seeking pain management for a particular symptom. She also told me that her gall bladder had been removed several years before. In fact several people in her family had had their gall bladders removed.

  I have proven for myself many times over that thought creates, so I seriously have to wonder what a person actually means when they tell me their symptoms run in the family. I tend to think more along the lines that thought patterns run in the family and eventually create a disease, or that family patterns suppress emotions which change form into matter.

  Either way, a gall bladder issue is connected to intense anger, bordering on rage. Addressing that sort of family pattern may have negated the necessity for an operation at such a young age.

- A woman came with a digestive problem. She suffered with chronic constipation, and her bowels wouldn't move without laxatives. She had recently been through a relationship break up and was putting much of the blame on her ex-partner. She seemed to be stuck in her emotions which appeared to be compacting in her bowel.

48

Respiratory System

I take in... I give out...
I administer the unseen life force
There is balance in my receiving and giving

Overview

The respiratory system is related to fair exchange and transition. It inhales your vital life force and exhales the residue. Your organs are energized by the transition that takes place with the air you breathe in.

Dysfunction of this system will draw your attention to an imbalance in your ability to give and receive. You must take in before you give out. Receiving is the primary action; giving is secondary, but one does not work without the other.

You may not be willing to receive because you have a feeling of unworthiness or not being good enough, beliefs brought with you from childhood. You may have been made to feel guilty because others in the world were less fortunate than yourself, or you may believe that if you go without, someone else will have more.

You have the capacity for receiving much more than you are aware of, or accept. There is an abundance to draw to yourself, but you will not always allow yourself to be filled up, for you have come to believe in lack.

You make many transits in your life as you pass from birth to death. For those you love who move too quickly and have left before you are ready to say goodbye, their transition can be felt in this system.

When you have a sense of being crushed and suffocated and find yourself fighting for breath, a breakdown in this system is showing you that you need to escape from the constricting effects of others. As a child you may not have been able to do that. As an adult you are able to make changes if you want to.

When you repeat the same words, thoughts and scenarios over and over in your head, a blockage in your sinuses is telling you that you need to take action, not just listen to the resounding of your own words.

Metaphysics of the Respiratory System

Respiratory Passages
Connected to a life-giving force

Nose
Sticking your nose into someone's business
Offering help when it isn't wanted

Sinuses
A resonance chamber for speech
Something is 'in your face' and needs to be dealt with

Pharynx
How well do I share

Larynx
Speaking your own words
Saying what others want to hear

Epiglottis
Knowing which way to go
Staying on track
Changing direction

Trachea
Hot air, all about nothing
Blocking your life force

Bronchi
My essence is intricate and delicate
Transition

Lungs
Constriction
Suffocating
Being over or under nurtured
Fair exchange
Crushed
Life force

Diaphragm
Automatic relaxation
Rest is vital to sustaining life

Messages of the Respiratory System

I am the see-saw
Weighted unevenly is out of balance
Fair exchange is the pivot

If your ability to give outweighs your ability to receive, you need to consider what you believe about give and take.

Unbalanced giving can be a substitute for low self-esteem. If you don't think you will be liked for who you are, you can make sure you are respected for what you do, and give to extremes.

Your need to be received can be so intense that people take advantage of you.

Before you stick your nose into something, gauge whether your comments will be welcome.

While Spirit is your essence, you may not always turn to it to renew your vital energy. From where do you draw your life force, and how do you feel when it is cut off?

As you wheeze and struggle for breath, who is suppressing your breath of life.

There comes a time to speak up and say what you need to say, or stop thinking about it, and take action. Allowing negative thoughts unrestricted access to your mind is draining.

Take notice of your words and what you say. They could well be reflecting your own thoughts, but they may also be conforming to what someone else expects of you.

It takes wisdom to know when to change direction in life. The dilemma is to know the difference between a temporary block, needing to persevere, and hitting your head against a brick wall in frustration.

When you pay attention to your life you will know which path to follow. When you don't, you may need some firm redirection to put you back on a more direct pathway.

Some exchanges rest on a delicate and fragile balance.

51

Over-nurturing your children can be a cover for possessiveness and control. When your self-worth is connected to parenting, letting go of your children so that they can lead their own lives can be threatening, leaving you with a sense of emptiness.

Consistent and repetitive relaxation needs to be part of your everyday lifestyle. You can always find excuses. You do have time. It is your priorities that need to be rearranged.

Example

- A client came with infected sinuses, but then many people come with sinus problems. My first thought about sinuses is that they are a resonance chamber for speech. This woman couldn't think of anything that kept going over and over in her head. There was nothing that was in her face that she needed to deal with. A few weeks later she told me she had left her partner.

Urinary System

I monitor, clean and recycle
I know about perfect balance
I rejuvenate and reuse

Overview

The urinary system clears the body of waste, regulates the amount of water, and balances the components in the blood. It knows exactly how much to keep and reuse, and how much to let go.

This system is your gauge of how well you have taken what you have learnt from one situation and applied it to another. It knows what is useful and needs to be taken forward into the next cycle, and what has reached its use-by date. It knows how to refresh the tired and exhausted with energy and vitality, and put it back to work. It has the wisdom to know what is of no further use and the courage to release it.

You may find discomfort in this system when you come to retirement age, believe you have nothing more to offer in the workforce, or you are unable to find employment with which you are happy.

When under stress, it can be trying to tell you that a situation needs to be neutralized before you do irreparable damage.

Metaphysics of the Urinary System

Kidneys
Monitoring a situation with the intention of taking action
Keeping the balance
Knowing what is useful and what is out of date
Decisions to be made

Ureter
>Very slow progress
>A little at a time
>Wanting to get something over and done with
>Impatience

Bladder
>Holding back
>Storing up and keeping count

Urethra
>Release

Messages of the Urinary System

Retirement came and I wasn't ready
Surely my working life can't be over
I still feel strong and able
But youth is no longer on my side
Oh! that the wisdom of my years will arise
And a new world find me

Before you remove something from your life be sure to recognize what its purpose is and if it has been accomplished. There is a wisdom attached to knowing what stays and what goes.

Close enough is sometimes not good enough.

Balance is the key that brings harmony and accord. Balance is the secret ingredient that has everyone working together producing positive results.

Monitor your actions and behaviour. Assess the situation regularly. Make adjustments as you recognize a need. If you leave it too long the correction may be overwhelming.

Difficult decisions are part of life. Not everybody has the courage to make them. Often they are ignored, hoping they will resolve themselves.

You may need to take up a neutral position.

You can learn patience from the impatient if you can see them as a teacher and not an obstacle.

When you are always in a hurry, you will miss the finer details of living. Some things just need a little more time.

There are many ways to eliminate waste and residue, always with gratitude for what they have taught you.

Such pain and agony in holding on when you know you would be more calm and comfortable letting go. Recycle your pain to enrich your future.

You may be able to see potential when the other can't, and you may need to encourage them to continue with their pursuits.

Example

- An elderly gentleman was introduced to reflexology by his daughter who regularly gave him gift vouchers. He didn't have kidney disease himself, but his wife had been on a dialysis machine for some years. Eventually, her health failed, and she died. A few months after her death, he developed kidney disease, and found himself in the same hospital, with the same staff looking after him as when his wife was still alive. Unlike his wife, the dialysis treatment was temporary. After a few months, he was back to his normal healthy self, and the kidney failure was just a memory. He had been devoted to his wife and it was as though he was deciding whether to go with her or to stay behind.

Reproductive System

I reproduce
I create new life
I express creativity

Overview

The reproductive system is your gauge and willingness to express your creativity.

In the years gone past, it was often said that a woman's place was in the home. Children, husband and home were the only acceptable means of self-expression a woman could choose. Modern times are different. A woman's role is to creatively express herself.

Dysfunction of the reproductive system occurs when creativity is shut down in one way or another, sexual urges are repressed or fear of self-expression is given into.

Women who have never expressed who they really are get a second chance at menopause. It literally is an invitation to change their lives, and divert their creative energy into something new. Ignoring the invitation to change can bring with it uncomfortable symptoms.

Men, on the other hand, can experience problems in this system as they grow older. As younger men replace them in the workforce and they feel they are being set aside or 'shafted', the ability to be assertive fails and symptoms appear in this part of their body. If retirement brings with it a sense of being cut off and isolated, they may find their prostate gland will react.

Women who are slow or unable to conceive, and men who have problems with sexual performance could be working with the Universe on a level that the conscious mind cannot recall or understand. Children or intimate relationships may be a distraction to their life purpose in this particular lifetime.

Metaphysics of the Reproductive System

Female
Ovaries
Maturing process
Blocking creativity

Fallopian Tubes
Starting a journey
New beginnings
Joining together

Uterus
A safe haven
Developing my creative skills
Beginning new projects

Vagina
On the move
Joining the real world

Breast
Support and nurture

Estrogens and Progesterone
Defining femininity

Male
Testes
Fighting for my place
Competing
Passive aggression
Swimming against the tide

Prostate Gland
Choked
Strangled
Cut off

Semen
Mobility
Ease of transfer

Penis
    Delivery
    Being shafted
    Set aside

Testosterone
    Defining masculinity

Messages of the Reproductive System

I am your gift to the world
Something created deep within you
Something hiding, waiting for expression
Only you can bring me forth
I wait in hope for the gift of you to emerge

You are not in competition with anyone, ever, because no one does anything the same way you do. Everyone is so different; there is no scale for comparison.

Confidence and creativity go hand in hand. If you don't develop one, you won't bring forth the other.

Aggressive pursuit might make you the leader, but what cost did it incur?

While you might need respite from time to time, you eventually have to live in the real world.

First impressions leave an imprint which can be a misrepresentation. First thoughts might need to be changed. The wise person has his second thoughts first.

Learn where the line is drawn between support and control, nurturing and possessiveness.

When you ask someone to do something, let them do it their own way.

Maturity doesn't always align with age. Be prepared. It pops up suddenly in unexpected places.

Example

- I remember a woman who was trying to become pregnant and found that she had endometriosis. She said that it had spread so quickly she almost thought she created it herself. Both husband and wife were eager to have a child, so what could be an underlying reason to sabotage a pregnancy. It wasn't hard for her to find the answer. If she had a son, she would have to name him after the paternal grandfather who had the same name as her previous partner. There was no way she would be able to do that.

Integumentary System

I am the boundary that defines you
The visible expression of all that you are
The touch, the sensation
Perpetual renewal

Overview

When you have a problem with your skin it is more than likely that your boundaries are being stretched, and you are being forced out of your comfort zone. You may be on show for something you have created, or noticed as you stood up to be counted and found yourself alone.

When you take short cuts through a process your skin can tell you that you are trying to avoid the necessary steps.

Skin is the indicator of how well you insulate yourself from a situation or another person. If you don't like someone to touch you, especially your feet, you are giving a clear message that others should keep their distance and respect your space.

The more skin you show, the more you give the appearance of being open, but that can be misleading. Your openness might only be superficial, the real you might never surface for others to see.

Metaphysics of the Integumentary System

Skin
Epidermis
Thick skinned
First line of defence
The brush off

Dermis
"You've got a hide"

Subcutaneous tissue
Locked in place

Skin appendages
Sebaceous glands
Blocked pathway
Softer approach
Sweat glands
Cool down

Hair
Something that can be done without

Nails
Impractical approach
Focused inward
Self-centred

Messages of the Integumentary System

I am your cloak of protection
The shield of all that is fragile and delicate
A versatile robe for you to wear
I stretch, I flex, I bend, I reach out, I extend
Come with me

Before you can extend your boundaries and reach new territory, you actually have to travel to them. You have to gather your courage, face your fears, push at what confines you, and make a break through. You can't explore new ground from your comfort zone.

Your mind is the most intense boundary you have. Opening to new thoughts can mean closing off old ones. Some don't leave readily.

You'll never be able to stretch yourself unless you take your mind with you.

Skin can be a way of releasing emotional toxins to make space for the new.

Personal growth is a cycle with several steps: learning, processing, assimilating and moving on. Gathering information is of little use unless you do something with it and experience the result. Letting it sit as theory won't extend you.

Appearances can be deceiving. What you see is not always what you get.

Everything will penetrate overly sensitive thin skin, but thick skin might keep the best out.

Your ego can disfigure the real you. What image are you trying to live up to?

Examples
- A woman who was extremely negative had come to see me over a long period of time. She wallowed in self-pity and blamed everyone for what didn't work in her life. This was one of the few times when my boundaries of tolerance were really being stretched. I asked the Universe to take her permanently out of my diary. She developed a skin problem on her feet, and rang to cancel her next appointment. She never returned.

- A lady came to see me because her skin had suddenly broken out in a rash. I suggested that it could be something about extending her boundaries or being on show. She didn't think either of those issues applied to her, but she did tell me that she had recently entered her garden in a competition, and she was concerned as to whether it would be good enough. She also wondered what her neighbours would think. She was absolutely sure her skin problem had nothing to do with putting her garden on show.

Special Senses

I cross all time and space
And take you with me
I make you feel as though you are reliving the experience
What is real and what is your imagination
You must decide

Overview

Special senses are essentially a part of the nervous system, and are therefore connected to how you collect, process, interpret and assimilate information. Memories seem to have a special place with the senses: seeing something beautiful can stir your heart to a smile, hearing a certain song can transport you to a special time and place, taste can immediately bring to mind what you like and dislike, smell holds such strong recall that it can bring on a physical reaction, touch can be as gentle as the evening breeze or hold the fury of a hurricane.

Metaphysics of the Special Senses

Eyes
    Do you have vision or simply see
Ears
    Hearing is different to listening
Taste
    To touch, estimate or judge
Smell
    To "smell a rat or something fishy" is another way of saying "a deeper awareness has been activated"
Touch
    To heal or to hurt

Messages of the Special Senses

I hold your memories
I keep them safe
I tuck them away somewhere
and
your mind forgets
Until they are stirred once again
To be as real as they ever once were

You may unknowingly suffer with tunnel vision and only be able to see your own point of view.

Are you so focused on a specific that you can't see the obvious?

Do you listen with the intention of understanding, or do you only hear?

When you finally get the message, the next phase is action. Sometimes, it is better not to hear.

Once you hear something, you can't unhear it.

Just a little taste will tell you if you are about to bite off more than you might like to chew.

Your body is led by the nose in more ways than one.

Touch is indelible and felt much deeper than the skin.

Examples

- I could have put this story in a few places, but because it is about weeping, I'll put it here.

  An elderly gentleman had suffered with a weeping ulcer on his leg for fourteen years. His relatives thought that reflexology may help with circulation, and eventually the ulcer might heal. I asked if anything in particular had happened fourteen years ago. Nothing came to mind. In the course of the conversation he told me that his wife had died fourteen years ago. Her death coincided with the time the ulcer began. His stiff upper lip approach to life didn't allow him to weep for her, so his leg did it for him.

- This is another eye story that comes to mind.

A lady came along with a weeping infected eye. The tear duct had been blocked for almost twelve months. All attempts to heal it were unsuccessful, and a date had been set for an operation. She came along with the hope that reflexology would relax her in preparation for her hospital visit. Of course, the eye healed, and she never underwent surgery.

Six years before her eye problem she had a mastectomy. She was dedicated to her own family and the mother image for her siblings. I don't think she ever stopped and wept for herself after her operation. She felt everyone's pain but her own. I think her eye wept the silent tears from her own loving heart.

Holistic Reflexology Principle # 2
Chakras reveal flow and blockages in energy

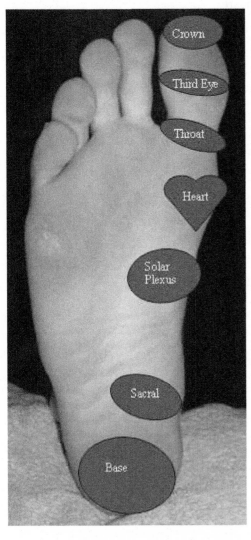

Chakra energy takes us through a transformation from our most basic primal instincts in the base chakra to our highest spiritual self in the crown. Reversing the process, it brings back what we discover in the spiritual realm, and keeps us grounded and practical in our everyday living. It applies a higher perspective and a greater understanding to our lives, bringing a calmness of purpose and a knowing that everything is exactly where it is meant to be at any given moment.

When I look at a foot I don't focus on the toes, skin or bone structure. My foremost interest isn't the physical reflexes. I am more concerned with the issues attached to a specific part of the foot.

When I look at the heel, representing the base chakra, I think about family and beliefs. The lower arch and soft tissue extending to the ankle reflect the sacral chakra and direct my thoughts to relationships, money and power games. The upper arch, the solar plexus, will have me considering personal boundaries. The heart chakra sits on the inside ball of the foot and draws my attention to love and forgiveness, joy and happiness.

I see the base of the big toe as the most complex area of the foot, the throat chakra. It is the crossroads, the pivot between the heart and the head, the signpost to the past or the future. It holds responsibility for speaking up and consciously creating your own life circumstances.

Midway up the big toe I find the third eye chakra, the place of judgment, where something is made right or wrong. At the top of the same toe is the crown chakra, embracing all that is involved in connecting to Spirit.

As we open to this energy and flow, we might describe ourselves as growing. When we block the information coming to us through these energy vortexes, we may think of ourselves as stuck.

Base Chakra

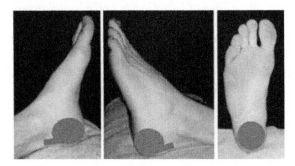

The base chakra energy is needed to ground you, and hold you secure in this physical reality. However, you can have such a false sense of security in the physical that you do not seek the spiritual. When you are able to ground your spiritual energy, and put it to work for you in a practical way in your everyday life, you will create for yourself a lifestyle of choice rather than being encased by circumstances for which you accept no responsibility.

The base chakra is where your basic instincts reside: the survival skills that will keep you safe, the secret behaviour patterns that rule your life, your deepest and confirmed beliefs, and your reactions that can sometimes surprise even yourself, as they sit in waiting, ready to rise up and defend you in an instant.

An un-evolved base chakra isn't particularly interested in a higher purpose. It is primarily interested in survival, one of the strongest forces in nature. It will often compromise potential to achieve this end.

This same chakra embraces the ancestral heritage you were born into: the groups, cultures, traditions, religions, beliefs and genes. It holds what your families and generations before them followed or belonged to. Your ancestors or the tribe, as it is often called, can be dictatorial. You need to honestly assess whether the beliefs of the tribe encourage and support your higher purpose and potential. If not, you need to consider the alternatives.

The challenge of the base chakra is to decide if you still belong to the tribe, or where you stand in relation to it. Also to be considered is what you have done, or what you continue to do, to survive there. You also need to assess the appropriateness of the survival techniques you use in your everyday life.

Issues

Your relationship to the group
Your place in relation to the family, tribe, society, tradition or culture
Family dynamics (parents and siblings)
Childhood
Your emotional security
Your ability to integrate into the community or group
A sense of not belonging or not feeling part of something
Religious beliefs and cultural traditions
Rules of the group that must be obeyed
Family beliefs that you have inherited
Basic survival instincts
Behavioural patterns and habits
Reactions rather than a choice centred response

Healing the Base Chakra

On some level of your consciousness you have allowed, created or drawn to yourself your own reality. Everything is your own creation.

You have a life purpose that you chose before you came to the earth. Take some time to search for it. Astrology is an informative tool.

You chose all of the circumstances that you birthed yourself into. Why do you think you made those choices, and what are the strengths you have learnt about yourself through your family?

Let go of having to have an answer. There are many things in life that can't be explained in the moment. Wisdom unfolds slowly. How many times have you heard it said, "In retrospect, that was the best thing that could have happened to me?"

Refuse to blame anyone for what is happening in your life. You are not a victim. You are the one in control. Whether you believe it or not, you do have a choice. All too often it is more comfortable to hold on to what you know, rather than venture into the unknown.

You are exactly where you are meant to be and your life is on track, even though it may not make any sense at the moment. Logic thinks it has all the answers, but it doesn't.

Value what you have created and be open to its lessons. If you run away from them, they will follow you and show up in a different place in another way.

Make changes to your inherited beliefs if they do not serve your highest purpose, and draw forth your greatest potential. Muster the courage to leave the group if you know you have to.

Re-evaluate the cost you pay to belong. Acknowledge how much of yourself you compromise to be accepted.

Ground your spiritual beliefs. Put what you learn to work for you in a practical way. Apply what you learn from personal development, reading, life experiences and meditation to your everyday life, and you will change.

Acknowledge that living in a community or society requires guidelines to maintain stability. There are some rules for the good of the whole that need to be respected.

Recognize your behavioural patterns that keep you locked into survival mode. You need to know what beliefs and patterns run your life before you can begin to dismantle them.

Love the earth. Take care of it. Be environmentally aware.

Position
   Heel area

Reflex
   Lower spine, pelvic area, sigmoid colon

Examples
- A lady came to me with a right sore heel, with pain travelling up the heel and across the soft tissue towards the ankle. The pain began in base chakra and travelled up to sacral chakra area. My first thought about the foot pain was that it was something to do with a group or belonging issue (heel) which continued on to some sort of money concern.

   This lady had been regularly seeing a podiatrist for many months and wearing orthotics. Nothing was giving relief, and an operation seemed to be the only option left to relieve the pain.

   Her husband was a minister of religion and was close to retirement, which meant they would leave the area, their friends and their home of many years. They would relocate, be estranged from everyone who had supported them in the past, and re-establish their life. They would soon be leaving the community in which they both played a vital role. Like many people facing retirement, there were concerns about future finances. She understood the connection I was making between her foot pain and her forthcoming lifestyle changes.

Before long she was back driving, walking, exercising and doing all the things she hadn't been able to do for many months. She was also acknowledging the emotions associated with this change of lifestyle. There was never any more talk of an operation.

- A young woman came with digestive problems resulting in a distended stomach which became more intense when she exercised. The stomach area of the foot relates to the solar plexus which is foremost about boundaries. She told me she felt quite limited in the job she did and wanted to do something more creative. She said the job contained her when she knew that she had greater abilities.

The stomach reflex wasn't particularly tender. Her plantar heel area was close to unworkable, which made me think about other issues. The 'something more creative' she wanted to do was to have a child but that posed a problem. She and her husband had come to Australia to find jobs and save money. They hadn't achieved their goal as yet and weren't ready to return to their homeland. They didn't want their children to be born and raised in Australia without the broader support of their families. The plantar heel was telling the story: her place in relation to her homeland, family and finances.

Sacral Chakra

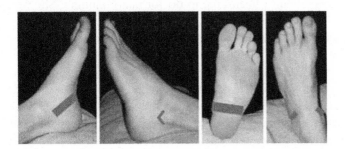

Once you become disillusioned with the tribe, you begin to move away, but all too often you are not strong enough to stand alone and immediately look for another tribe or group to belong to. You can move from tribe to tribe and relationship to relationship for many years, looking to others for support and strength.

The sacral chakra energy will help you to discover yourself as an individual if you understand how it works. You will only learn about yourself in relation to someone or something else. When relationships are unpleasant you may not recognize yourself in the other person because you are focusing on the negative and what they are doing to you. In contrast, if you were able to recognize a situation as a learning experience and focus on what you were learning, some of the more painful relationships would be understood in a totally different light.

Many of the intense learning and growth experiences break down into power games and a struggle for supremacy because you don't understand that you set them up in the first place to learn about yourself.

Again, you can mistakenly think that a good relationship is your life's goal when in reality it is only a means to an end, discovering who you are.

When you finally realize that your sense of belonging, your security and your rules come from within, you eventually learn to stop looking to others. You realize that it is the relationship with yourself that is paramount. But until you find yourself, you will search outside yourself for the answers to life.

Issues

  One to one relationships
  Your ability to connect with others
  Sexuality
  Creative expression
  Gathering and depending on material possessions for security
  Money
  Power games
  Manipulation
  Aggressive competition
  Using people

Healing the Sacral Chakra

Everyone in your life is a reflection of you in some way. What they reflect back to you is foremost your issue, not theirs. The other person will share a core issue with you, but may express it differently to the way you do. If you focus on the expression of the core issue that this person has brought to your attention and not get to the underlying commonality, you may never understand what it is.

You have created everything in your life for a higher purpose. Are you not grateful? Nobody does anything to you without your permission on some level of your consciousness. As long as you are focusing on what the other person is doing to you, you are missing a valuable lesson.

Nobody is trying to hurt you. When someone is 'pressing your buttons' they are trying to get your attention, and help you identify something in your life that needs to be addressed. They are bringing up a particular issue for you because you are not able to begin the process yourself.

All relationship lessons are to teach you something about yourself which is a positive and a strength. If you want to move through a particular lesson as quickly as possible, focus on yourself not the other person.

If you try to understand the world from a logical perspective, the pain and suffering you find may overwhelm you. Be aware that it is your own pain and suffering to which you are connecting. You need to identify it and begin to address it.

Let go of your jealousy and competition. We are all here for different reasons. No one is in competition with another because no two people are the same. My uniqueness is equal to your uniqueness. Complement the other rather than compete with them.

Let go of your greed for there is enough for everyone. The problem is not shortage. You may discover that one of your primordial beliefs, hidden deep within, is that you are not worthy and therefore do not deserve. Another of your beliefs could be that there is not enough to go around, so you must grab more than your share to survive.

Let go of your belief that material goods will bring you peace of mind. Consider how many times the stock market has crashed and how many people have lost their fortunes. Ultimately, what you believe about money is your security, not money itself.

Looking outside of yourself to find meaning for your life will not give you the answers that will satisfy you and bring you peace of mind.

Sexual obsession can be the distraction you require to escape your journey to self. You can allow passion and desire for another to fulfil your needs, when in reality nothing outside of yourself can do that. Intimate union can become your goal rather than a means to an end. You can merge so deeply with another that you lose your sense of self-identity.

Position
The sacral chakra sits slightly higher up the plantar surface of the foot than the base chakra and extends into the soft tissue of the lower arch and over to the ankle.

Reflex
Hips, gonads, lower back

Examples

- Client presented with plantar fasciitis on the right foot, around the sacral chakra area with pain moving across the soft tissue towards the ankle. The symptoms had begun two months previously, but the client had suffered with it before that time as well. She clearly remembered the circumstances surrounding her first attack. It was related to her sister, who was unmistakeably the matriarch of the family. My client's feet eventually settled down but only if she wore a particular brand of shoe. Her feet were pain free until two months before she came to visit me when another incident erupted with her sister. Once again for a second time, the pain was instantly back in the sacral chakra area of her foot. The power games had begun once again.

74

- A woman came with a painful right ankle. She and her husband were about to retire and lose their incomes. She had great concerns about their finances.

- Two women, both of whom suffered with irritable bowel syndrome shared an almost identical family situation. They were both the matriarchs of the family and were key players in the family dynamics, not surprising that it showed up in this part of the body.

Solar Plexus Chakra

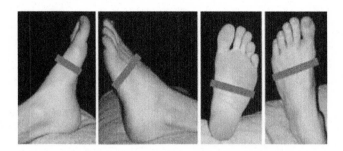

The solar plexus energy will establish and define you as an individual. It will enable your being and disable your compulsive doing. This energy introduces you to choices, confirming that you always had them, even if you didn't realize you did.

Your whole being will be energized when you honour yourself. Putting yourself first may not be clearly understood by those around you and explained as selfish, but it is essential to your future health and wellbeing.

Others who are not on the verge of discovering themselves may not give you permission to take this next step. They have depended on you to give them security and keep them safe. They have used you in their power games and dramas, so they would not have time to look more deeply at what life is intrinsically about. You will find resistance all around you.

The entrapment of what you should be doing will be cast like a net from every direction, but you are strong enough, committed enough and determined enough to continue.

Logic may present you with the personal cost of this giant leap to self, trying to convince you that it is too high a price to pay. Emotional attachment at gut level may churn you to the point of not knowing which way to turn.

You have moved from loyalty to the group, through loyalty to another and arrived at loyalty to yourself.

Issues

Your relationship to you
Personal boundaries
Liking and honouring yourself
Your rules and integrity
Self-respect and self esteem
What you should be doing
Imposed guilt
Pressure to conform
Gut feelings

Healing the Solar Plexus Chakra

Acknowledge the necessity of putting yourself first. It is not selfish. It is essential.

Clarify your personal boundaries. You may discover that you have no boundaries at all, and others just walk all over you with their demands and expectations. You may think you give to others, when in reality, they blatantly take from you.

You may have built brick walls around yourself to keep everyone out. You may only feel safe when you hold others at a distance.

State the new rules you intend to introduce which will change how you prioritize yourself. Make rules that honour you and your needs. Remember you do have needs.

Define who you are and put yourself on show. Others may initially react, but it is only because you are no longer playing the same old game. It may take some time for them to adjust. Be patient. You are moving into an awareness that they may not understand.

Get to know yourself without judgment. Discover your likes and dislikes, your dreams and hopes, your strengths and weaknesses, and use it all to your advantage.

Get to like yourself, then you will honour yourself, and keep your commitments to yourself.

Develop self-loyalty. Make promises to yourself and keep them. Be your own best friend, and treat yourself as such.

77

Be honest with yourself. Look at reasons, not excuses. You are past hiding from others and especially from yourself.

Be a person of integrity and let your actions match your beliefs and words. People notice integrity. It draws great respect.

Discover any old belief patterns that don't support and value your self-worth. Then release them with gratitude, for they no longer have a place in your life.

Stop listening to other people and voices in your head telling you what you should be doing. Everything you are told you should do carries with it guilt, and guilt is nothing more than pressure from an outside source to make you conform. Guilt is an emotion cast upon you to try to force you to change your priorities.

Take time out. Relax. Take respite from your life circumstances. Concentrate on being, rather than doing. Give yourself permission to make changes. Others might not.

Position
The solar plexus chakra sits in the soft tissue of the upper arch

Reflex
Stomach, small intestine, pancreas, liver, gall bladder, lower thoracic spine

Examples

- A client came with an aching upper arch on the left foot. I ran my fingers around the foot at the point and said, "That's the boundary band."
  "I've divorced my mother." she replied.

- A woman came who had suffered with sore feet for the past two years. She wore orthotics, and blamed the floors she walked on. Her left arch was painful while her right foot was hot with the discomfort extending to the knee. The initial problem began when she retired, and family expectations came thick and fast. She needed to put some boundaries around her newly acquired spare time.

Heart Chakra

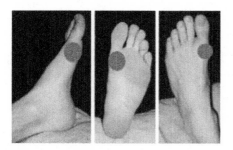

The energy of the heart chakra beckons you to celebrate who you are. You have reached the point in your evolution where you know, without any doubt, who you are and what your life is about. There is no emotion or thought attached to knowing. It just is.

A vibrant heart chakra merges logic, emotions and basic instincts to an indefinable knowing, a knowing that urges you to follow. You no longer need to understand everything, and you are no longer are controlled by emotions. You simply know. And that knowing will lead you in safety to wherever you choose to go.

Everything is embraced, as forgiveness is transformed to gratitude. You understand there was never anything to forgive, for everything was your own creation to learn about yourself. Everything has always been on your terms.

You expand with gratitude for the person you were, the person you are and the person you are becoming. You are touched by the perfection of all that is. You know your life is exactly where it is meant to be. As you celebrate the gift of yourself, you cannot help but celebrate the gift of others.

The knowing energy of your heart is the catalyst that will push you forward, and help you to manifest a life of choice rather than one of unrelated circumstance. You are not afraid to love. You open your heart to others. You invite them to share your great treasure.

Who I am, is no longer challenged by who I think I am.

Issues

Joy and happiness
Compassion and gratitude
Love, hate and forgiveness
Self-nurturing
Conditional love
Martyrdom

Healing the Heart Chakra

Make choices that bring you joy and happiness. Mix with people who help you connect with those same feelings.

Let your inner child play. Allow your creativity to be expressed and appreciated.

Be grateful for your perceived failures because they enable you to become more compassionate. Happily embrace them because, in reality, they were intrinsic life lessons you needed to experience.

Forgive yourself. Your life is exactly as it needs to be at this moment in time.

Love yourself unconditionally. Stop finding fault with what you look like, what you do, or how you express yourself. Be glad to be you.

Observe what conditions you attach to your love. Do you feel someone owes you something or needs to repay you because you once were good to them? Have you ever said, "After all I have done for you!"

Over-nurturing your children is often associated with a person whose self-worth comes from motherhood or fatherhood. Clinging to children, under the guise of protecting them, could be your way of not opening your heart to possibilities for yourself.

When you listen to the wisdom of your heart, you will discover what is best for you. It doesn't mean that you know what is best for someone else.

Recognize a difficult lesson someone has set up for themselves, and try not to destroy it. They will only have to set it up again. Distance yourself a little from your logic and emotions, and know all is well.

Position
The heart chakra is found on the inside of the foot, near the bunion joint where the skin changes colour and thickens.

Reflex
Heart, diaphragm line, part of the lungs

Example

- One client travelled constantly and lectured, an amazing woman. I could only work on the balls of her feet in a certain way because they were so sensitive and touchy. The rest of her foot was fine. A broken relationship, along with a forgiveness issue for a parent sat in her heart chakra, while grief for the same parent resided in her lungs.

Throat Chakra

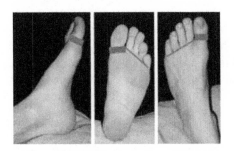

The throat chakra is the energy for creating your own life circumstances through conscious choice, rather than existing within unexplained chaos. Underpinning the power of your words is responsibility.

Before you can consciously draw to yourself circumstances that you choose, you must accept responsibility for everything in your life. If you are not responsible, then it follows that someone is doing something to you, and you are powerless. When you know you are in control, you have the power to make changes.

Responsibility is the key issue of the throat chakra. You are only responsible for yourself. You disempower another when you take responsibility for them.

The creative energy of the throat chakra, like everything else in the relative universe, has a positive and a negative. If you want to manifest a positive outcome, you must think and speak positive thoughts and words. If you are not able to control your thoughts and are constantly thinking and speaking negatively, then a negative result will follow you wherever you go.

To empower the throat chakra to create by conscious choice, you must realize another two things. The only place is Here and the time is Now. Many people are not able to live in the Here and Now reality. We all take short trips away from it, but for the greater part, we need to stay there.

The throat chakra is the pivot point of Here and Now. We also use this point to swing between the past and the future. The throat energy is negated by living in the past, because the good old days were so much better. Alternatively, you can move away from Here and Now into the future, where everything will be better once a situation has changed.

If you are not guided by the knowing of your heart, the imbalance between the logic, gut feelings and survival instincts will show up in this area as well. While the battle between these three rages for dominance, the throat is powerless to create anything by conscious positive choice.

The throat chakra energy gives you the power to express your inmost authentic self, speak up, claim your innate ability to create, manifest your dreams and transform your life.

Issues
Speaking up
Creating your own reality by conscious choice
Battle between the logic, gut feelings and survival instinct
Living in the past or projecting to the future
Responsibility
Powerlessness

Healing the Throat Chakra

This is the point of balance between passive and aggressive. Peace at any price is not peace, and aggression is not always appropriate. This is the point to speak with assertive conviction, and change your reality.

Speak with truth and integrity. It is the greatest power you can yield. Listen to the wisdom of your own heart, and let others know who you are and what you believe.

Make your own choices, and accept responsibility for what they bring to you. You do have a choice. You have always had a choice. You may not have known it.

Be aware of how you respond. Does your mind hold the power over your actions? Do emotions carry you into situations that you would prefer to avoid? Do you react with an instinctive survival response? Can you hear the knowing of your heart which can appear like a flash of lightning from nowhere, and be gone again in a moment if you do not hold on to it firmly?

Take the time to recognize the beliefs and thought patterns that have dictated your life experiences. You have to know what they are before you can change them.

It is easy to change a belief. Once you have learnt how to control your thoughts, you will learn how to create a life of conscious choice.

Notice the words you use to describe your circumstances. Notice if there is a connection between what you say and what you see appearing in your life.

Let others be responsible for their own choices. They have created their circumstances to learn from them. If you don't allow that from a compassionate perspective, they will just have to keep re-creating them until they learn.

Visiting the past is one thing, living there is another. Use it to move forward, rather than hide there. Don't be too quick to crave for the future. The future may not happen as you expect.

Position
The throat chakra is found at the base of the big toe

Reflex
Cervical spine, referring to the shoulder

Examples

- A client presented with a stiff neck. It had only been a problem for a few weeks. She couldn't think of anything that she was being inflexible about. We stood at the door and chatted before she left. I wished her all the best for the holiday she was about to embark upon. She would be away for a while and needed lots of clothes. She couldn't understand why her husband was objecting to her taking so many pairs of shoes and outfits. There were many dinner parties to attend on the cruise and tours, and she didn't want to have to wear the same thing twice. Even though her husband would be the one carrying all the cases, the subject was utterly non-negotiable.

- The right side of a lady's jaw had been painful for the past two years. She had tried everything, and reflexology was her final attempt to see if she could find some relief. I wondered if anything in particular had happened about the time her jaw became sore. Of course, her brother had died. His death was something that she hadn't been able to talk about to other family members. Not so strange that the pain settled in her right jaw. She talked about him during the whole session. The pain went away before she left, and it didn't return.

- A client presented with an irritating throat condition. It had been a problem for many years. She never knew when the next bout would attack her. This woman received quick and amazing relief through

84

reflexology and as the weeks passed, she began to tell me many things about herself. There was a particular family situation that she wanted to discuss with her husband but had never found the courage. She recognized the underlying cause of her condition and chose to do nothing. Her symptoms returned worse than ever within a few months.

Third Eye Chakra

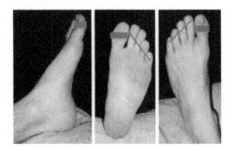

The energy of the third eye will take you past the physical, the logical and the explainable to an understanding of the metaphysical, the unseen and the esoteric. This energy is the doorway to all that you are, the portal to all that is not held within your conscious memory.

The third eye invites you to move through the three dimensions of the physical world into a realm of possibility. It offers you an opportunity to understand yourself and life in general, from a different perspective.

The third eye will open to you your psychic connection, that non-physical force that explains spiritual phenomena. This energy connects you to the spirit world and many profound secrets of life. It brings to the fore the collectiveness of who and what you are, and enables you to access and apply that information in the physical world.

The world is evolving and we are evolving with it. Times are changing and we are swept along. The shift is from the Age of Pisces, an age where we listened to wisdom from outside of ourselves and followed in trust, to the Age of Aquarius. This new age is connected to the mind and understanding. No longer do we have to follow another in trust. We have the ability to listen to our own inner wisdom and follow because we understand.

Issues

Seeing from a different perspective
Making something right or wrong
Judging
Psychic abilities
Other dimensions
Closed mind
New ideas

Healing the Third Eye Chakra

Understand what is happening in your life rather than accept it in blind faith.

Distance yourself from a specific, and see it from a different perspective. Open your mind to possibility, and look with vision not focus.

Let go of your previously held explanations which didn't bring you satisfaction, and start afresh. Look past the physical with the intention of seeing what is not obvious.

Acknowledge the positive and negative balance of the physical Universe. The value systems of many groups and cultures have changed this essential polarity to right and wrong. Right and wrong are not definites. They are relative to a specific value.

Refuse to judge, allow things to be as they are. Refuse to judge yourself, and you will learn not to judge others.

Open your mind to your own psychic abilities, everyone has them. Some people have developed them more so than others. It's your own choice whether you use them or not. In many ways they are your own personal short cuts which will bypass the long and tedious labours of the mind and logic.

Consider life forms and realities outside of what you can see and explain. The mind may accept angels and loved ones who have passed on, but what else and who else shares this universal plane with us.

Let go of the fear that holds your mind fixed and closed. Opening to new concepts is not being disloyal to what has gone before. New information is constantly around you. It is a positive trait to process anything new rather than dismiss it unexplored. Change is a constant. Anything that doesn't change in some way is usually dead. Don't let your mind ring your death knell by refusing to consider change.

Position

The third eye chakra is found at the base of the nail on the big toe

Reflex

Nose, jaw

Examples

- A lady came along to relax. Her nose reflex was very touchy, painful to the extreme. I wondered if she was sticking her nose into someone else's business. I asked was she offering advice which wasn't being readily accepted. Her partner had made a decision without including her in the negotiations and possible outcome. It was non-negotiable. Maybe she just had her nose out of joint.

- A woman had a strong frontal headache, just above her eyebrows, for several weeks. She understood how I thought, so when I asked what happened a few weeks before, she instantly recalled an event. She had asked her husband to do something for her. He did it his way, not her way and the headache hit almost immediately. As far as she was concerned he had done the wrong thing by her. He didn't consider for a moment what she wanted and wouldn't see it from her perspective.

- A client came along with painful toes. She had been bedridden after a particular illness several years earlier, and during the recovery process had been advised to wear orthotics which she had done until four weeks before she came to see me. She felt her feet had become stiff because they were held so tightly in place. That was exactly what I thought when I met her, so contained, except for her eyes. She had beautiful eyes. It was as if they sang and danced for her, while she maintained a stoic pose. She didn't speak much during the session, nor did I. She didn't appear to have any interest in the way I thought, but she did say her feet felt good when she left. Besides the usual notes I took, I wrote "This free spirit needs to be free!"

  She returned six months later, a totally different person. There was no sign of the rigid one I had met previously. During those months she had twice gone back to the country where she was born, and had set up a business which was doing very well. She was about to leave again in a few days. This time the balls of her feet were sore. I asked if there was anything she was feeling guilty about. She was very concerned about leaving her elderly mother once again, the amount of money she had been spending, and how great her life had become.

Crown Chakra

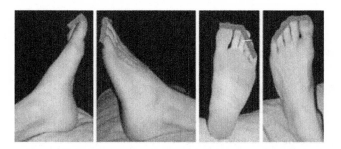

The crown chakra is the doorway to your innate spiritual nature. Its purpose is to dissolve the ego and unite with spirit. It seeks to break down the barriers of illusion, so you can understand the oneness of all creation.

As you allow its energy to transcend from the higher realms into your physical reality, it has the ability to transform you. As you embrace what you know in spirit, and apply it to your everyday life in a practical way, you will understand the meaning of grounding.

As the energy of the crown descends down through every cell of your body, you become humbly aware of the opportunity it brings with it for change.

- The smallness of the logical mind is opened to possibility.
- The insignificant voice speaks with authority and creates a lifestyle of choice.
- You respond to your heart guiding you with knowing and wisdom.
- You honour and respect yourself.
- You acknowledge all those around you as your teachers.
- You are grateful for every physical experience because you understand that it was all on your terms.

The crown makes sense of the past, shows hope for the future, brings understanding to the chaos, and casts peace and calmness wherever it moves. You are left with a sense of knowing that all is well.

Issues

Unity and Oneness
Illusion
Universal guidance
Closure
Transformation
Self-mastery
Ego
Fear of the unknown
Control and trust

Healing the Crown Chakra

Know that the Universe and all that it contains is perfect. Life is unfolding as it should.

There are no mistakes, accidents or coincidences.

Trust Spirit to guide you. Take absolute control away from your mind, logic and ego.

Accept the reality of your own life with gratitude, rather than live in the illusion of how you would like it to be. Escaping the disillusionment, disappointment and confusion of the world is done in many ways.

Some things must end or close to allow something new and refreshing to enter.

Look at the world through the eyes of Spirit. Not a lot makes sense when you only see the physical. Trust when you don't understand, and wisdom will eventually show herself.

Boundaries protect and contain you at the same time. Know the difference, and push through those that limit you.

Your vision is short. You can only see to the horizon. To know what is beyond, you must first visit it.

Your ego is the ultimate boundary. It holds you firmly attached to the things of the world.

When the ego dissolves you are able to live in the physical and spiritual world at the same time and connect to others with compassion as one.

Your ego is necessary to define you but it can separate and ostracize you from others at the same time.

Position
The crown chakra crowns the top of the big toe and extends out along the tops of all the others

Reflex
Brain

Examples

- A client came on and off over several years for reflexology treatments, but she seemed to be more interested in all the other courses and energy work I was doing. As a rule, we would spend the session chatting. Whatever questions she asked me, I would answer as truthfully and openly as I could. She seemed interested, yet wary, and obviously stretched beyond her comfort zone more than once.

  She told me she wanted to try out the Reconnective Healing™ I was doing at the time, but had read enough about it to know it would change her in some way. She was well connected to a group of more traditional business women, and she knew they wouldn't be open to some of the things we discussed. If she changed, she wasn't sure how these women would accept her with her new ideas.

  I can still see her face as she asked me in all seriousness, "How do you feel when people think you are mad?" She obviously thought I was mad, yet intriguing at the same time. She was looking for that last piece of information so that she could decide if she would open up to a more esoteric approach to life. Before she left on that particular day, she decided that she would rather have the friendship of the women's group than continue with any spiritual ventures.

  The following week she returned. She said she felt like she had a concrete cap covering the top of her head since the previous week. No wonder. She had not only decided to cement her relationship with the women, but she had closed off any thought of conscious spiritual movement for the present moment. No wonder her crown chakra was bringing pressure to her head.

Holistic Reflexology Principle # 3
Elements express their energy through the toes

I remember a drawing I saw when I began to study astrology. Two men, who looked like Greek philosophers, were standing in front of a blackboard, appearing to be having a discussion. On the board were four words: air, earth, water and fire. One of the men was pointing to them, and the caption said, "What do you mean, it's a start? That's it!"

The Universe is comprised of those four elements, though Aristotle added aether to the system of the classical elements and named it the *fifth element*. There isn't anything else. That's all there is. There is nothing more. Everything and everyone, including you and I, are a combination of these elements. What makes it all so amazing and interesting is the ratios of definition. The sun, a rock, a flower and a person are all different combinations of the same elements.

My understanding and interpretation of the elements is closely associated with my knowledge of astrology. Each toe has its own energy.

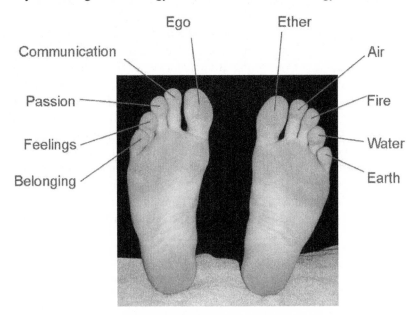

ETHER expressed through the big toe embraces the oneness of creation.

Ether is more associated with the spiritual realm than the physical one, but I have included it as I see its role as being somehow connected to holding the four elements in suspension in this physical reality of earth.

Ether is your passage to all that is not of this material world. It transfers you through the elements to Source. It brings you to a knowing that is beyond time and space, logic and understanding. Ether is the essence of being. It simply is.

AIR expressed through the second toe is connected to communication, which is nothing more than an exchange of information dependent on how you think and analyze.

Communication is expressed through:
- the intellect and transfer of data
- beauty, the arts, relationships and justice
- the visionary ideas of the humanitarian and scientist

Air is of your mind, and focuses on ideas to be understood, and ideals to be materialized. It changes direction so often, you can't always keep up. It needs stillness to allow it to slow down. It gives you the ability to express your innermost beauty with integrity, honesty and honour, or allows you to simply say what others want to hear.

FIRE expressed through the third toe is associated with passion. When your passion for life and all you do has diminished, you simply exist.

Passion is expressed through:
- initiating your own ideas and making them happen
- expressing your own creativity
- expanding your horizons by travel, adventure, learning or philosophy

Fire is your energy and impulse to be a leader who spontaneously and fearlessly steps into the unknown. Fire can be so passionate it wants to take others with it, whether they want to go or not. Fire can consume you and destroy you at the same time.

WATER expressed through the fourth toe is related to your feelings. How you feel about yourself defines how you relate to others.

Feelings are expressed through:
- emotional connections and nurturing of others
- reaching deeply into the powerful and invisible emotions far below the surface with the intention of transformational change
- unity and oneness for humanity through compassion

Water allows you to connect with others through feelings. Its compassion and empathy can become somewhat sacrificial if it doesn't respect its own boundaries. It has the ability to connect so deeply that it can be possessive, intimidating and unrealistic.

EARTH expressed through the fifth toe is linked to grounding and belonging. Earth is something to be seen, touched, heard and sensed. It needs the tangible to be secure.

Earth is experienced through:
- producing and consolidating something tangible by patience and persistence
- being of service to others and offering practical help
- authority, responsibility, commitment and your public image

Earth is where your roots are planted, where you came from, your origins, your survival instincts and your inherited patterns. Earth holds you in a time and place, and provides your culture, religion or belief system. It defines the group, the tribe and the family tree. Your sense of belonging comes from the earth.

Examples

- A female client told me that every so often the second toe on her right foot got very sore, but only when she wore a particular pair of shoes which was once every week. I wondered why she wore these particular shoes each week and what was she doing when she had them on. I was beginning to think that the problem was connected to communication with a male.

   She was a teacher of sorts, who shared this teaching role with her partner. She was the leader and taught six nights of the week. She didn't really want her partner to teach at all because she didn't like his method, but she let him teach just one night a week so he wouldn't feel left out. That one night was the night she wore the shoes that gave her a sore toe. She never commented on his teaching methods because she knew it would erupt into an argument, so she kept her mouth shut, didn't communicate what she really felt and thought, wore the same shoes every week and blamed the shoes for the sore toe.

- A client presented with a Morton's neuroma which I think of as a communication issue usually going nowhere. His toes caught my interest. His third toe was protruding and the fourth toe curled underneath the third.

  I began to think about a work related issue, something he was passionate about but because the fourth toe was tucked underneath it, he lacked confidence in whatever it was. The Morton's neuroma was telling me that there was a communication issue around the whole event.

  I basically said that to him and he didn't respond. Twenty minutes later he told me about his work situation. He had developed something noteworthy in his workplace. His efforts were not acknowledged. Another colleague took credit for it. The client was devastated at what had happened and resigned. He had recently gone back to the original place of work because he knew he had to deal with the situation, and not run away from it this time round.

  By applying my holistic principles to his toes, I could tell him, in summary, his own story before he told me anything.

- Second toe on the right foot was raised up and painful. The client's intention was to get the toe to sit back down in line with the others. I suggested this could be a communication issue with a male. She began talking.

  At the end of the session she told me that she had revealed more about herself to me in that one hour than she had to anyone she'd ever spoken to before. I don't try to solve clients' problems, but it never ceases to amaze me that if they speak about them, they usually see them from a completely different perspective. All I do is give the starting point and an opportunity to talk.

- Client with a noticeable separation between the second and third toe, air and fire. She had a lot of good ideas, but wasn't able to follow through and make them work for her.

Holistic Reflexology Principle # 4
Organs hold emotions, often suppressed

Emotions play a vital role in drawing your attention to a situation. They are a beam of light that focuses on a particular issue. They are the beacon of the lighthouse that can be understood in two ways: dangerous area, keep out, or safe passage continue through to calmer waters.

Your emotions will rise in an instant as a first and automatic response. What you do with them is secondary. Whether you choose to feel them or suppress them, is a choice. You can shut them down within micro seconds of their appearing, or you can choose to allow them to direct you to a deeper issue that needs attention.

As it is usually another person who helps you raise them, all too often you concentrate on what that person has done to you, rather than benefit from what has happened.

As long as you are immersed in an emotional response to any situation, you will never get to the positive lesson it holds for your own personal growth. Working through your emotions may take years. It may never happen at all. You have a choice. You can hide in the positive, wallow in the negative, or be guided to what needs your attention.

Emotions are intrinsic to human nature and must be acknowledged. If you choose to suppress them they will settle in your body, and make their presence known in another way. Each emotion has its own special residing place within the body.

When you are able to accept responsibility for every situation and acknowledge that on some level of your consciousness you gave permission, emotions can be processed more quickly. They can be seen for what they are, a highlight to something about yourself that needs addressing.

They are also an accurate gauge indicating when you have dealt with a given situation.

I have not studied Traditional Chinese Medicine in depth. I have only cast a passing glance, during an adult education course, over a couple of months.

As with everything else I have explored, I take a few basic principles and work with them to see if the results are consistent with what I expect them to be.

The organs that take my interest are the liver, kidney, lung, heart and stomach. There are several body parts and functions associated with each of these organs, but I tend to only take notice of a few.

I have consistently found grief and guilt to show up in the reflexes of the lungs. Grief tells you that you should have been given more. Guilt tells you that you should have given more, and forces responsibilities upon you that aren't yours to carry. Responsibility at an early age can hold the forefoot in dorsiflexion.

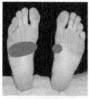

Liver emotions: anger and resentment
Body tissue: tendons and nails
Sensory organ: eyes

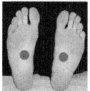

Kidney emotions: fear, terror and phobia
Body tissue: bones and head hair
Sensory organ: ear

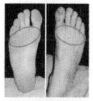

Lung emotions: grief and guilt
Body tissue: skin and body hair
Sensory organ: nose

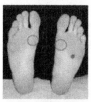

Heart emotions: joy from agitation or overexcitement
Body tissue: blood vessels and facial complexion
Sensory organ: tongue

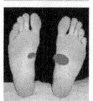

Stomach emotions: anxiety and stress
Body tissue: muscles and limbs
Sensory organ: mouth and lips

Examples

Kidney:

- I once had a client who belonged to a motorbike club. One particular night, working her kidney reflex just about put her through the roof, but she didn't have any kidney problems.

  The day before the treatment she had been on a long bike ride. For some reason she had left the group and rode home on her own. She kept just in front of a wild storm the whole way. The sky was dark and threatening, and she eventually got caught in the rain. Reports the next day said trees had been blown over and property damaged. She said the experience terrified her.

  I have no doubt that the fear she experienced settled in her kidney reflex for a short time. Not to forget that the adrenals would have been well overworked at the same time, but the intense pain was lower than the adrenal reflex.

Lungs:

- A long term client has had a chronic lung disease for many years. Her lung reflexes are often painful as is her solar plexus area. Two of her children were born with disabilities. Her young son died some years ago and her daughter, who still lives at home, requires full time care. Her lungs are the obvious place she would carry the grief for her children.

  She works in a support unit for families with disabled children. Needless to say, her commitment to the needs of others, because of her own first hand experiences, drives her in her work. She needs to put a few boundaries in place so that she is not on constant call for all who need her help. Slowing down a little might help her solar plexus chakra to settle.

  She told me the reason she has continued to have weekly reflexology treatments for the past seven years is that she believes it is the main reason she has been able to minimize her stays in hospital.

- A woman presented with swelling across the dorsal surface of the right foot proximal to the base of the toes. I think of that area as the back of the lungs. I began to consider grief in relation to a male, which goes hand in hand with guilt and responsibility.

  There were substance abuse issues in relation to her son and she was involved in a battle for her grandchildren. She was not only grieving for her family but had also taken on responsibilities which were not hers to carry.

- A young woman came for reflexology to assist her asthma condition which she had developed at the age of eleven. Eventually, she recalled that her much loved dog, who was her best friend, died when she was eleven. She had never connected the dog with her condition. The adult was still holding the grief of the child in her lungs.

Heart:

- An older woman had experienced a breakdown in the relationship with her adult child over many years. All attempts at reconciliation only left both parties and the broader family even more distressed. The relationship was the cause of deep unhappiness. Passing each other by was the best way to deal with it. She had a heart bypass operation.

- A middle aged man married for many years didn't appear to be happy in any way. Disappointment had been a part of his life for many years, the world owed him. It was as though happiness had passed him by completely. He also had a bypass operation.

Stomach:

- One particular person I remember only came to see me when she was extremely stressed. She knew she needed to relax, but would never close her eyes. She talked incessantly about what was going on in everyone else's lives but hers. I presumed her anxiety was related to her work which kept her very busy. She was obese and blamed her weight on stress. She told me she would stand at the open fridge and eat. I asked her what she was thinking about when she did that. Surprisingly enough she wasn't thinking about her work, she was thinking about an elderly family member who wouldn't do as she said.

  As long as her problem was stress, it was an all encumbering fog, but once it was identified, she could begin to address it if she wanted to.

Holistic Reflexology Principle # 5
Left and right define who, how and when

I began with the limited understanding of right equates to male and left to female. From there I expanded the feminine and masculine traits to arrive at a broader interpretation of definition through left and right. This principle helps me to find who is involved, how it unfolds and when it happened.

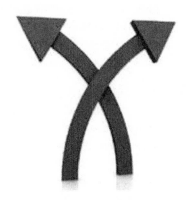

Who
Left: feminine, female, women
Right: masculine, male, men

How
Left: being, unconscious, intuition, nurturing, passive, spiritual, mother principle
Right: doing, conscious, logic, supply, aggressive, physical, father principle

When
Left: present and future
Right: past

The left and right principle is usually combined with other information I have observed to give me a clearer indication of the situation causing the discomfort. I would use more intuition with this principle than any of the others.

For example, if the solar plexus chakra on the left foot was tender, I would suggest there may be a boundary issue with a female. Alternatively, a painful sacral chakra area on the right foot could be telling me about power games in relation to a male. I often find that the left heel is related to the mother and the right heel to the father. Siblings will often show up in this area as well. I tend to suggest a broader group rather than pinpoint a specific person. Usually the client will quite readily expand the story.

Examples

- A lady came to see me with a left ankle problem. Several operations had not improved the ankle, and she felt the problem was back where it all started. As an afterthought, she told me that the fifth toe on her left foot was swollen and tender. She thought she had broken it. Also as an afterthought, she told me that she had cared for her father for many years, and he had died recently. She had been very close to him.

  The toe drew my attention before the ankle. The toe had been sore for about eight weeks, and her father had died eight weeks before, but she had not put the two together.

  The father's illness and death would have shown up on the right foot. The left ankle and toe were most probably related to the mother. She told me her mother was still alive and had become more and more difficult over the years as focus was given to the father.

  As the ankle is the reflex for the hip, which is associated with power games, and the small toe is related to belonging and family, the foot problem clearly was related to the mother. What was going to happen to her now her husband had died? The left ankle was related to the client's future in relation to the mother.

  The client came back the following week. Her small toe was back to normal. There was no redness or pain.

  "I don't know what you did," she said. "You hardly touched it." All I did was bring her attention to the underlying cause.

  Not every time I lead someone to the underlying cause will it heal. Sometimes it does, sometimes it doesn't. I don't try to figure it out.

- Female client presented with Morton's neuroma on the left foot which I suggested might be related to communication issues with a female. The client confirmed that two females in the family were very strong women who had a great deal of influence over her husband. Her right foot went into cramp when I worked the solar plexus area, indicating boundary issues relating to the husband. He wouldn't hear a word against these women. His defences were up, boundaries set and no discussion allowed.

- Single male client aged in late thirties presented with a left lateral ankle problem. He had fallen when on holidays six months

101

previously and his ankle was still painful. MRI ten weeks previously showed no tear, chip or break. The ankle was normal to walk on but if he turned or twisted, he felt as though he had no strength in it. The client couldn't remember any particular incident happening in his life at the time of the accident.

He was a particularly gifted and skilled person, and had held several creative occupations over the years. He was also passionate about an unusual hobby which he had set up in depth at the family home, even building an extension to the house to contain it.

When he came to see me he was looking to change his occupation once more to something he had always wanted to do. He was thrilled about the new job offer. He had completed an exhaustive application process and had passed with extremely good results, except for the medical examination which he couldn't undertake because of his ankle.

The ankle was the only thing standing between him and his new job. It was the barrier, the block. He had to discover what it represented. What was his block to the new job? What reservations did he have? Why was he holding back?

When the ankle was presented in that context, he could immediately see what the problem was. The hobby he was passionate about was the issue. There was a strong possibility that he would be transferred to a country area which would cut him off from the family home where the hobby had been established. He couldn't take it with him and further involvement would be impossible at such a distance. He felt if he accepted the job as offered, he would have to give up his hobby which was a major part of his life. That's why I believe it showed up on the left not the right. It was about creative expression, not doing a job.

To resolve the ankle, he needed to negotiate with the new employer regarding where he would work.

Holistic Reflexology Principle # 6
Shape, texture and position show strength and weakness, potential and challenge

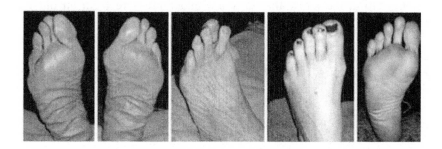

I'm sure this is a principle that most reflexology practitioners would follow whether they are interested in metaphysics or not.

It is surprising how many people I've met who don't like their feet. Very few comment on how nice their own feet are. Also, most people live with the illusion that feet naturally have an unpleasant odour. I rarely wipe a client's feet before I work on them. To me, wiping their feet is like putting them into a sterile environment where I will miss the messages that the feet are trying to convey. The way you think about and appreciate your feet has a lot to do with how you think about and appreciate yourself.

At first glance there is usually something that literally jumps out at me. The general shape and proportions will tell me if a person has an overall balance to their life.

Calluses and thickened skin are obviously some form of defence, and where they sit on the foot points to what they are protecting.

Deep cracks and splits around the heel indicate a breaking away or splitting from the group, family or tradition.

Spurs or protruding bone shows that something is being restructured or fortified.

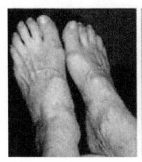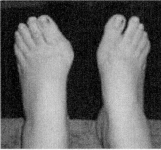

Bunions at the heart area of the foot talk to me about stoic resolve. As the tendon slips and the heart protection weakens the bunion develops as strong protection.

Blisters are letting me know that they are under pressure from an outside influence.

Plantar warts, unlike other warts, are sensitive to pressure. They are usually found on the plantar surface of the ball of the foot or heel, a sign of sensitivity to the family or heart.

Infected nail beds imply that something is eating away at them.

Ingrown toenails can suggest focusing inwardly on yourself or being self-centred.

A crunchy texture at the top of the toes is suggesting that the person spends a lot of time in their head thinking about things.

Sprained ankles with torn ligaments and tendons lead me to think about relationships and money issues.

Lateral base of hallux holds many secrets, one being whiplash. They have been whipped back to have a second look at something, or they have been given a great push from the back to get on with it.

Dorsiflexion with protruding tendons has repeatedly shown me a person who has been given responsibility at an early age or, as an adult, something had been thrust upon them that they felt they had no choice but to take up.

Toes that are curled under draw my attention to a person who can be stubborn and won't be told anything. They continue to do everything their way even to their own detriment.

Shape

One interesting shaped foot had a very high dorsal arch which fell away to a floppy mass, as if she had risen to every occasion and then collapsed. One such foot belonged to a woman who had run after everyone for many years, never stopping for a moment to nurture herself. She eventually had a double mastectomy. She did change her lifestyle.

I worked with a lady for a few years who was in her nineties. In her younger days she had been a brilliant musician, a lead violinist in a prominent orchestra. She stopped playing when she had a child.

When she returned to her music, she was offered a place in the orchestra. She told me that if she couldn't be lead, then she wouldn't be part of the orchestra. She wanted to be remembered as the best. She never picked up her violin again. By the time I began working on her feet, all of her toes were turned under. She had dug her toes in (as the saying goes) and never played again.

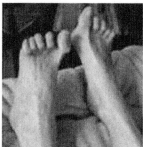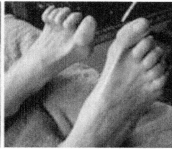

Texture

A woman in her thirties presented with low energy. She was concerned about her recent weight gain of 9 kilos. She walked daily, ate well and drank plenty of water. She was the mother of a young daughter and had miscarried two years before which still brought tears to her eyes as she told me. The texture of the uterus reflex was puffy and swollen, as if she was in late pregnancy. She wasn't pregnant. She was grieving.

One of my long term clients has a chronic lung disease. For the first twelve months or so of treatment her feet had a particular odour and an almost greasy feel to them. My hands would pick up the smell and hold on to it for a couple of hours after every session. The texture of her feet has completely changed as she continues to rid her body of toxins.

Position

A foot that refuses to rotate freely at the ankle, tells me that the person likes things done their way, and they are not very flexible in their approach to life. They want to hold their own position, and resist all else.

An upright foot tells me that the person knows what they want in life, and are well on the way to achieving it.

I've found that a foot falling outwards is trying to escape from something.

A foot that falls inwards wants help, is dependant on others and makes the person feel they literally cannot stand on their own two feet.

A foot that stands rigidly upright, stoic, tense and doesn't like to be touched tells me that the person is very protective of self and demands their own space.

I could count on one hand the number of people whom I have come across with ticklish feet. These people tend to be very sensitive in most areas of their life.

I have a client whose feet fall outwards to near right angles when she is dealing with difficult situations. When the issue is resolved both feet stand upright again.

With one client, I could work the left foot without any trouble but the right one was different. As soon as I touched the second toe, the third toe went into spasm. Every time I moved back to the left, the right toes would partially settle but as soon as I went back to the right, they cramped again. I said it could be about communication with a male. The third toe inferred work related. The client smiled. The foot couldn't have been more accurate. A major work related confrontation was scheduled for the following day.

Holistic Reflexology Principle # 7
Words and phrases draw a parallel to the cause

Paying attention is the greatest form of respect you can give anyone. It also allows you to pick up much more information than other people realize they are giving away.

The words people use to describe pain or symptoms are essential clues to the puzzle.

Those words are a paraphrase of what is happening and can often explain the underlying cause. You can also learn a lot from what is not said and what is passed over quickly as not relevant.

In my clinic situation I need to listen intently. Often clients are telling me the cause of their symptoms without knowing. They may not give me all of the information in the first few minutes but as the session progresses, I am usually told more of the story. The trick is to be able to put it together.

> I always ask two basic questions:
> How long have they had the problem?
> What was happening in their life around that time?

If nothing comes to mind, their feet will direct me to the next question. I absolutely know there is a connection. I keep asking questions or making comments until I find some common ground.

Some things I say may seem vague and irrelevant, but they are only meant to give them something to think about. I don't necessarily seek an answer to everything I ask. I just want to get people thinking. Often they will be quiet for some time, and then begin "Well... Maybe there was something..." and before long the story unfolds.

Words describing a symptom

One woman had severe pain on the inside of her foot where the lower arch meets the heel. She said, "It feels like someone is stretching it." Using her words back to her I asked, "Is someone stretching you?"

No answer. Actually nothing further was said during the whole of the session.

"Oops," I thought. "I must have said the wrong thing."

As the treatment finished and she stood up, she told me about how she was being stretched. How she described the pain in her foot told her story without her realizing it. The area of the foot, the sacral chakra, confirmed the power games.

Repeated words and phrases

A lady came to me who had been involved in an accident where several people had been injured. She had suffered severe damage to both feet. The metatarsals had been pinned but were now removed. The right ankle was still pinned, and tendon damage was in the process of healing, but with a good prognosis.

Her feet were very flexible, subtle and had good movement. The physiotherapist was obviously doing a great job. I began to wonder what she was doing in my clinic.

I began thinking about her words. When she phoned to make the appointment she mentioned the accident three or four times in the space of a few minutes, but only as a passing comment. Same during the session, she mentioned the accident several more times but again, only in passing. I began to wonder if there could be something related to the accident which had settled in her feet causing the ongoing pain.

"Wasn't someone killed in that accident?" I asked.

"Yes," she said as her eyes filled up with tears. "She was my best friend, and I was standing right next to her."

I felt we had finally got to what the foot pain was really about. Disconnecting from her good friend and restructuring her life with only her memory was consistent with tendon and bone damage.

Words describing an event

Often when a client speaks and describes something out loud, they will see the situation from a different perspective.

A pregnant mother came to see me. She had a little girl aged two and was expecting twins. She was constantly nauseous. Her mother suggested that a reflexology treatment may help her to relax.

"Just the thought of having twins makes me sick," she told me.

After a few more similar comments, I drew her attention to what she was saying. She said to me, "You sound like my mother, telling me to change my attitude."

"I'm not telling you to change your attitude. I'm merely repeating back to you what you are saying to me." I replied.

What you focus on you will create.

She came back a second time, feeling much more positive about the prospect of a larger family. Her nausea had left.

A middle-aged man with a long list of symptoms came to see me. He told me he had been very healthy until the day he retired.

"I was fine when I was working. I got sick the day I retired, and it hasn't stopped since. I knew the minute I gave up work, it would be all downhill from there!" That's how he thought, so that's what he created for himself.

A lady came for a reflexology treatment as she was recovering from an illness. She wanted to feel less tired and exhausted. Her husband had been sick for many years, but some time before, when she was ill, he got better. Then as soon as she recovered, he got sick again. This was the second time she had been ill, and her husband's health had improved. Now she was worried that as soon as she recovered, he would revert to his old illness. It seemed in her best interest not to improve her health.

Sometimes there are good reasons why a person will hang on to symptoms and illnesses.

When I was working on a female client she told me about her daughter who was allergic to nuts. She said that the thought of nuts made her daughter's mouth react. I suggested that if she focused on the thought of something making a change in her daughter's body, it would most probably happen.

She went on to tell me about an extended period in her life when she vomited every morning. She said the thought of having to get out of bed every morning, and do the ironing made her sick. Her husband and children stayed in bed while she had to get up an hour earlier and iron their school and work clothes. She used the word 'spewing', a descriptive word for when someone is furious and angry. Her feelings were so intense that they created a physical experience as well.

Holistic Reflexology Principle # 8
I attract my own issues

I attract to myself my own issues. That is a critical point to understand.

I bring to myself things about myself that need my attention and they are not always negative. It can be people and clients who have already developed my potential strengths who come to encourage me to do the same.

I will pull to myself groups of people with the same issues until I get the message the Universe is trying to communicate to me. As long as I keep ignoring the messengers, they will keep coming in some form or other.

The foremost reason I do what I do is to heal myself. That is the crux of it all. It is not about healing someone else. It never has been. It never will be. It has only ever been about healing myself. The same applies to you.

You also attract your own issues and bring to yourself things about yourself that need your attention. You will pull similar groups of people and experiences to yourself until you understand the message the Universe is trying to convey to you.

Messages come through your health, your career, your finances or your relationships. They can be a gentle whisper or a touch as light as a feather but if you refuse to listen, they will soon become a shout with the impact of a sledgehammer. I have learnt to listen.

Examples

- I had a run of women who were pregnant. That was in relation to drawing out my creative expression and writing a book, not this one, another one that took me many years to finish.

- I was going to pass through New York as a stopover until three women came in the same week to see me. All of them had recently been there, and all of them loved it. They couldn't understand why I would pass through and not even give it a second glance. I changed my plans. I loved New York.

- There was another group who came with very tender liver reflexes. I knew I didn't have a liver problem, so what else was my attention being drawn to. Anger and resentment reside in my liver. As soon as I said the word *resentment*, I knew exactly what my issue was. I had taken on a voluntary role which had consumed most of my time over many months. After working what seemed to be the equivalent of a full time job, I was feeling very resentful about the number of hours I had to put into the position to just maintain the basics.

  Once I was able to acknowledge resentfulness and connect it to a specific, I was able to do something about it. I didn't attract any more tender liver reflex clients.

- Before I began to study astrology, I made several unsuccessful attempts to find a teacher. My phone calls weren't returned, and I was becoming frustrated. I put it out to the Universe for a teacher. A long term client purchased a gift voucher for a friend, someone I had met several years before. In the catch up conversation, she told me she had been studying astrology for the past two years. The Universe had given me the information I had asked for.

Where to Next?

I love sharing my ideas, both the written and spoken word, so I was overjoyed when I was invited to be a speaker at the national conference of the Reflexology Association of Australia. In preparing my presentation, I realized I had so much more information than I would be able to use in the time span allocated to me. That was when I decided, against all odds, to put this book together and launch it at the conference.

Logic said that I would never pull it off as I had left it too late to begin, but the Universe stepped in, as always, and guided me to the perfect people I needed to help me achieve my goal.

I had written some of the content for a workshop a few years before so I thought all I had to do was expand it a little and put it together. Of course, that turned out to be a much bigger undertaking than I thought.

For a few weeks it became my total focus, for I knew that whatever I focused on expanded, and what I thought about with passion manifested itself in my reality. My energy also expanded as I sat for endless hours in front of my computer.

From my knowledge of astrology I knew that problems with communication can arise when Mercury goes retrograde. I must have focused too intently on that point because in the first few days of the project my computer crashed. I was never dissuaded from my purpose because I knew that the new moon in Virgo which is associated with health was passing through my ninth house of publishing. This was my promise that all would be well.

I had to smile to myself as I wrote the examples, and thought that I was telling the reader so much about myself by simply sharing the type of issues my clients brought to me. It was also interesting for me to remember when these groups of people came into my life and what was happening for me at the time.

While in the past I would have attracted people to challenge and draw my attention to what I needed to fix in my life, now I seem to draw many people who give me the most amazing snippets of information that are hugely beneficial to me and others. It never ceases to amaze me that someone can talk to me about something I have never heard of, and a few hours later another person is asking me if I know about exactly the same thing.

Writing now appears to be my next pathway of discovery. Before I began to put *Holistic Reflexology* together, I needed to put aside my other manuscript, *Wisdom in Retrospect*.

It had been two years in the writing, and was ready for proofreading and design. I wrote it because I found myself repeatedly talking about the same things to many of my clients. I began by writing down every profound learning experience I could remember and the year in which it happened. I could see immediately how my life fell into cycles of nine years. I could recognize what I had incorporated into my life and what lessons I needed to repeat. *Wisdom in Retrospect* is not meant to be my life story but sixty-four lessons of life I have learnt over almost as many years. Its focus is to help others make sense of the past, find hope in the future, understand the chaos and know that all is well.

But that is in the future, back to the present. I hope you have enjoyed reading *Holistic Reflexology*. I feel it is primarily about life, self-discovery and making your dreams come true. If you understand the messages your body is trying to convey, you will discover what areas of your life need attention. Many of those messages come to you through your feet.

May you look deeper into your symptoms, for they hold information yearning to be understood.

May you not just read the words, but take time to listen to what they say.

May you open your mind to possibility, for there is always another point of view to be considered.

May you be ready to embrace all that is new and challenging, for in doing so you may find the secret to the fullness of life.

Reflexes of the Nervous System

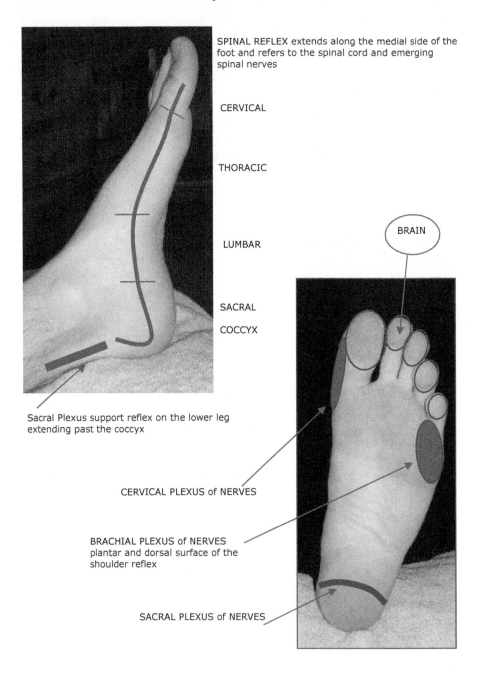

SPINAL REFLEX extends along the medial side of the foot and refers to the spinal cord and emerging spinal nerves

CERVICAL

THORACIC

LUMBAR

SACRAL

COCCYX

BRAIN

Sacral Plexus support reflex on the lower leg extending past the coccyx

CERVICAL PLEXUS of NERVES

BRACHIAL PLEXUS of NERVES plantar and dorsal surface of the shoulder reflex

SACRAL PLEXUS of NERVES

Reflexes of the Endocrine System

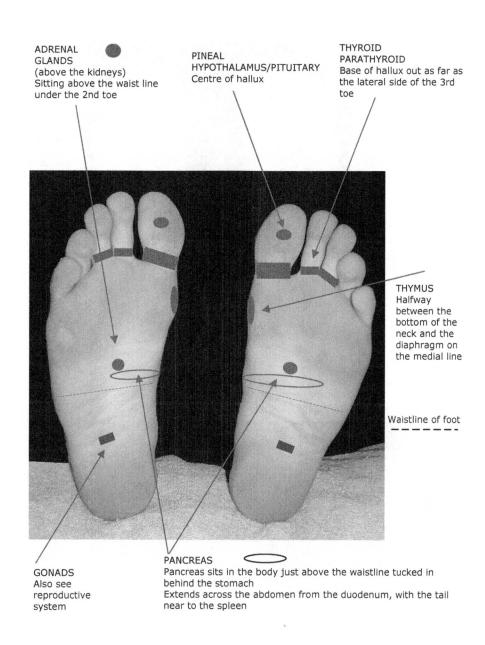

ADRENAL GLANDS
(above the kidneys)
Sitting above the waist line under the 2nd toe

PINEAL
HYPOTHALAMUS/PITUITARY
Centre of hallux

THYROID
PARATHYROID
Base of hallux out as far as the lateral side of the 3rd toe

THYMUS
Halfway between the bottom of the neck and the diaphragm on the medial line

Waistline of foot

GONADS
Also see reproductive system

PANCREAS
Pancreas sits in the body just above the waistline tucked in behind the stomach
Extends across the abdomen from the duodenum, with the tail near to the spleen

Reflexes of the Cardiovascular System

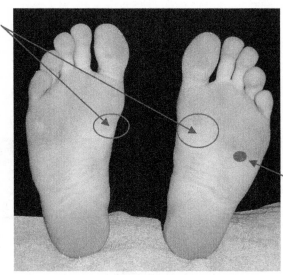

HEART REFLEX
Slightly bigger
on the left foot

The heart
reflex extends
from the
medial line of
the body on
and above the
diaphragm line

ORIGINAL
INGHAM HEART
REFLEX
and CHINESE
HEART REFLEX

Hook up under
4th toe on the
diaphragm line
on the LEFT foot

MAJOR ARTERIES and VEINS are found in the arms and the legs
and the center of the anterior trunk of the body

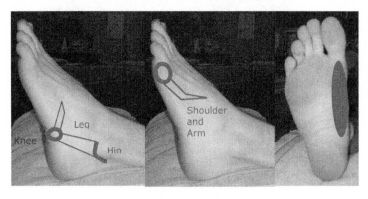

Leg

Knee

Hin

Shoulder
and
Arm

CENTRE of
ANTERIOR
TRUNK
Plantar surface

Reflexes of the Lymphatic System

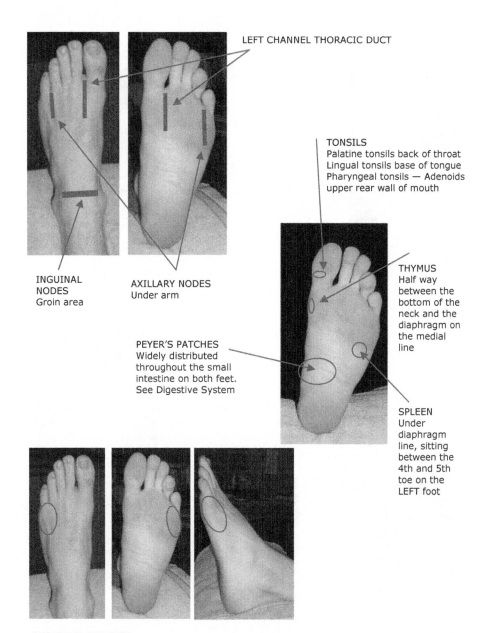

LEFT CHANNEL THORACIC DUCT

TONSILS
Palatine tonsils back of throat
Lingual tonsils base of tongue
Pharyngeal tonsils — Adenoids
upper rear wall of mouth

INGUINAL
NODES
Groin area

AXILLARY NODES
Under arm

THYMUS
Half way
between the
bottom of the
neck and the
diaphragm on
the medial
line

PEYER'S PATCHES
Widely distributed
throughout the small
intestine on both feet.
See Digestive System

SPLEEN
Under
diaphragm
line, sitting
between the
4th and 5th
toe on the
LEFT foot

SHOULDER REFLEXES
Work the dorsal and plantar reflexes and across the lateral foot

Reflexes of the Skeletal System

VERTEBRAL COLUMN

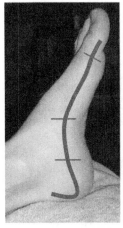

CERVICAL

THORACIC

LUMBAR

SACRAL

COCCYX

LEG
Extending in both directions from the knee reflex. Lower leg can sit in different directions. Look for tenderness in the area.

KNEE
Cuboid notch

HIP under and around ankle

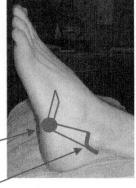

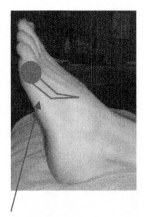

SHOULDER REFLEXES
Work the dorsal and plantar reflexes and
across the lateral side of the foot

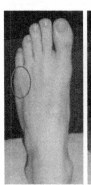 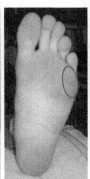 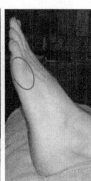

ARM extending from the shoulder reflex. Arm reflex can vary depending on how the arm sits on the foot. Look for tenderness in the area.

Reflexes of the Muscular System

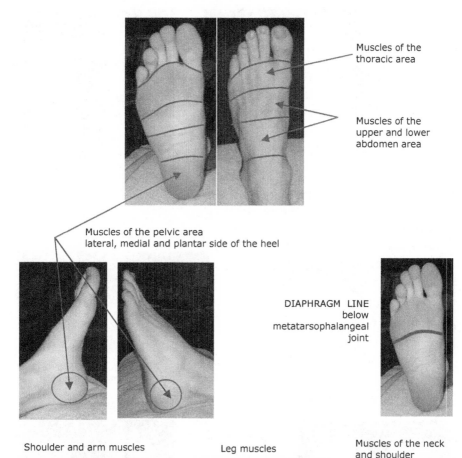

Muscles of the thoracic area

Muscles of the upper and lower abdomen area

Muscles of the pelvic area
lateral, medial and plantar side of the heel

DIAPHRAGM LINE
below
metatarsophalangeal
joint

Shoulder and arm muscles

Leg muscles

Muscles of the neck and shoulder

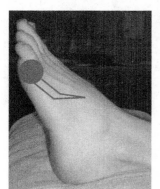

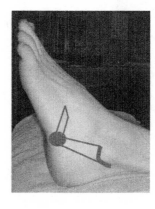

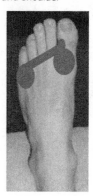

Reflexes of the Digestive System

GALL BLADDER sits in a shallow fossa towards the inferior surface of the liver

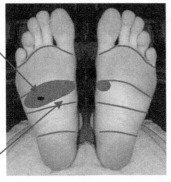

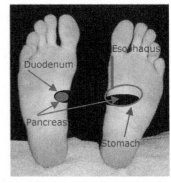

Esophagus

Duodenum

Pancreas

Stomach

LIVER
Tucks in under the diaphragm line and at the extreme right almost touches the waistline. The natural shape of the liver allows for the left lobe to begin on the right foot and extend over to the left foot.

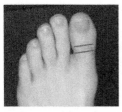

MOUTH reflex can be worked close to the jaw which is both sides of the joint of the hallux

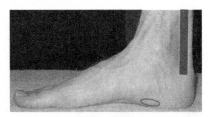

SUPPORT for CHRONIC RECTUM
Rectum follows on from sigmoid colon reflex

SMALL INTESTINE

LARGE INTESTINE

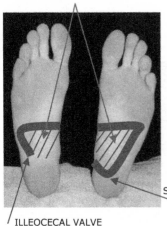

TRANSVERSE COLON

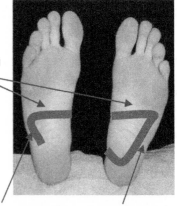

SIGMOID COLON

ILLEOCECAL VALVE

ASCENDING and DESCENDING COLON

Reflexes of the Respiratory System

LUNGS

PLANTAR   DORSAL

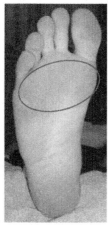
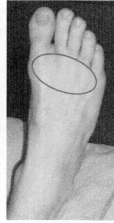

SINUSES
Pads of all toes and
working down 2/3 of
the toe

NOSE REFLEX
Under nail

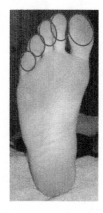
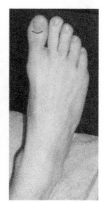

BRONCHIAL AREA
The right and left
primary bronchi are
formed by the division
of the trachea

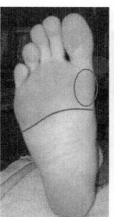
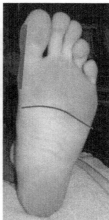

RESPIRATORY
PASSAGES
Pharynx
Larynx
Trachea

DIAPHRAGM LINE
Below the metatarsophalangeal joint

Reflexes of the Urinary System

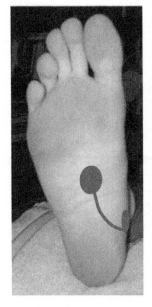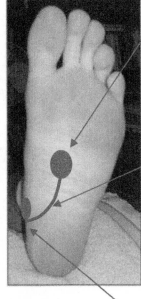

KIDNEY
The right kidney sits lower
in the body, tucking under
the liver

URETER TUBES
Flow out of the kidney reflex
down to the bladder

BLADDER and URETHRA

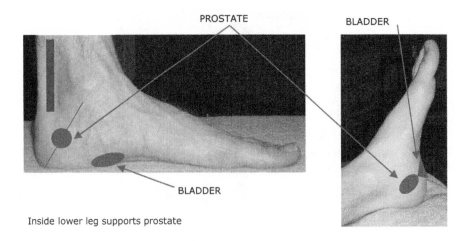

PROSTATE

BLADDER

BLADDER

Inside lower leg supports prostate

Reflexes of the Reproductive System

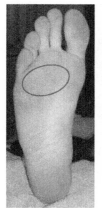 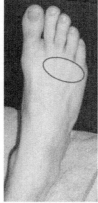

BREAST

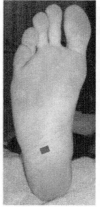 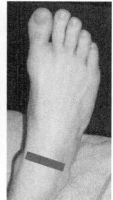

GONADS
plantar
surface

FALLOPIAN TUBES
between ankles

Outside Lower Leg   Inside Lower Leg
Ovaries   Uterus
Female issues   Prostate

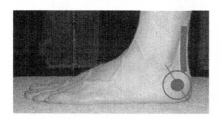 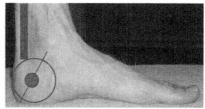

OVARIES
Lateral heel

UTERUS
PROSTATE
Medial heel

Reflexes of the Special Senses

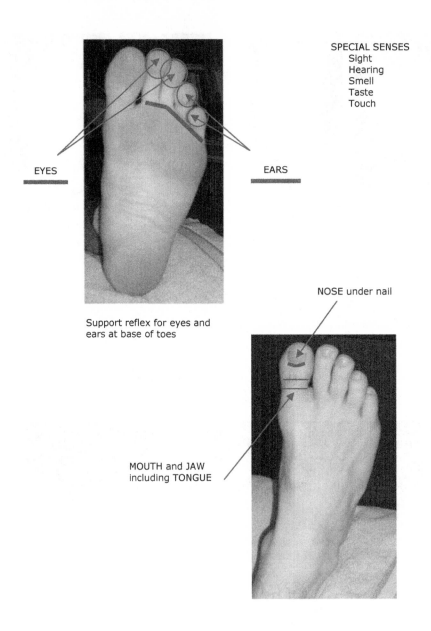

SPECIAL SENSES
Sight
Hearing
Smell
Taste
Touch

EYES

EARS

Support reflex for eyes and
ears at base of toes

NOSE under nail

MOUTH and JAW
including TONGUE

Afterthought

When the proof of *Holistic Reflexology* was at the designer stage, and I began to read it through, yet again, I realized that I had included a lot about what I believed, but very little about what I had done. Almost as an afterthought, I have included a few of the things that have kept me busy over the years.

2010   Dubai, my great escape.

2009   Dubai.

2008/9   *Wisdom in Retrospect*, 120,000 words, yet to be published.

2008   Designed a postcard with sixteen sayings related to all aspects of the feet entitled: *Everything I need to know about Life I have learned from Feet.*

2008   Federation of Australian Astrologers, Sydney Conference.

2008   Ann Arbor Michigan, New York and Dubai. -13° was a bit cold but the desert warmed me up.

2007   Self-published first e-Book entitled *Relax with Reflexology* containing over two hundred photos and diagrams which I compiled specifically for the home user. It was practical hands on information, and sold in Australia and America as a PDF file attached to an email.

2006   Self Identity H'oponopono Conference, The Foundation of I, Big Island, Hawaii. Facilitator Dr Ihaleakala Hew Len. I am responsibility. On some level of my consciousness I have allowed, created or drawn to myself everything in my life.

2006   Wrote and presented two workshops: *Relax with Reflexology* and *The Essential Foot*. This was a great learning experience for me. I was putting people into information overload.

2006   Psychic Development Workshops.

2006   Began to study astrology which is the most effective tool of self-discovery I have come across to date. My life purpose was captured at the moment of my birth, and by learning how to unravel its mysteries, I found a wealth of information to guide me along my pathway.

2006   Opened a local Chapter of the Red Hat Society, just for fun.

2006   Dubai in summer was hot.

2005	Chile, Argentina and Ushuaia, then back to Uruguay; climbing an active volcano and visiting Tierra del Fuego, the end of the earth.
2005	Orion/DNA Practitioner Course NLP Workshop Spiritual Surgery Workshop Channelling Workshop
2004/5	The Melchizedek Method: Levels 1, 2, 3, 4, 5.1, 5.2, 5.3, No Time Activation.
2004	Horstmann Technique: Practitioner Level Certificate.
2004	Reconnective Healing™ Self Mastery Conference, Sedona Arizona, speakers included Lee Carroll, Richard Gerber, John Demartini and Eric Pearl.
2004	Wrote and presented workshop: *The Dilemma of Forgiveness versus The Challenge of Gratitude.*
2002	The Next Evolutionary Step.
2002	Reconnective Healing™ Level I, II and III.
2001	International Council of Reflexologists Conference, Rome.
2001	Uluru. With respect we share the earth.
2000	Self employed as a Reflexology Practitioner, currently still practicing. Reflexology experience included my own practices, corporate offices, teaching staff, and the Sunday markets. I leased premises for a time, but I hadn't heard of due diligence and the adjoining shop was very noisy. After that I went on to rent rooms and work from home.
2000/5	Avid reader of new age literature.
2003	Peru, walked the Inca Trail to Machu Picchu. I didn't really know what exhausted was until I walked into the final camp.
2003	Thought Field Therapy.
2002	Chinese Reflexology. I began to change my style and use my knuckles.
1997	Self-published first book. It was a compilation of 270 of my own sayings entitled *Something to Think About.* I had written it for people, like myself, who wrote and formatted newsletters. I marketed the book to schools throughout Australia. The first few attempts weren't successful, but I quickly improved my sales letter and averaged forty-seven sales per hundred. A marketing course, which was the instigator of the book, was of great benefit to me.
2000	Reflexology Association of Australia, Hobart Conference.
1995	Ireland, London, Greece and Israel. This was the beginning of major change. I don't think the family believed I would go until I got on the plane.

1993	Catholic Parish Secretary for seven years.
1998	Reflexology Association of Australia, Brisbane Conference.
1998/9	Certificate IV Reflexology, Reflexology Academy of Brisbane. Reflexology I, II and III, Therapeutic Communication, Anatomy and Physiology, Nutrition, Aromatherapy, Swedish Massage, Professional Practice and Supervised Clinic.
1997	Reiki Level I and II.
1984/93	Domestic Manager/Housekeeper of a 200 bed nursing complex. This gave me the opportunity to expand my catering skills.
1967	Married and withdrew from the workforce. My numerous volunteer roles taught me many skills and prepared me to return to the workforce in 1984.

CPSIA information can be obtained at www.ICGtesting.com
Printed in the USA
BVOW08s0101240316

441445BV00002B/145/P